IBS

A self-help guide to feeling better

Wendy Green

Foreword by Dr Nick Read,
chair of The IBS Network

PERSONAL HEALTH GUIDES

IBS: A SELF-HELP GUIDE TO FEELING BETTER

First published in 2010 as *50 Things You Can Do Today to Manage IBS*
Reprinted 2013
This edition copyright © Wendy Green, 2016

Vie Books is an imprint of Summersdale Publishers Ltd

Summersdale Publishers Ltd
46 West Street
Chichester
West Sussex
PO19 1RP
UK

www.summersdale.com

Printed and bound by CPI Group (UK) Ltd, Croydon, CR0 4YY

ISBN: 978-1-84953-807-7

Substantial discounts on bulk quantities of Summersdale books are available to corporations, professional associations and other organisations. For details contact Nicky Douglas by telephone: +44 (0) 1243 756902, fax: +44 (0) 1243 786300 or email: nicky@summersdale.com.

Disclaimer
Every effort has been made to ensure that the information in this book is accurate and current at the time of publication. The author and the publisher cannot accept responsibility for any misuse or misunderstanding of any information contained herein, or any loss, damage or injury, be it health, financial or otherwise, suffered by any individual or group acting upon or relying on information contained herein. None of the opinions or suggestions in this book is intended to replace medical opinion. If you have concerns about your health, please seek professional advice.

To my husband, Gordon – thanks for being so supportive

Acknowledgements

I'd like to thank Dr Nick Read, chair of The IBS Network, for taking time out of his busy schedule to write a foreword.

Thanks also to Jennifer Barclay for commissioning the original book and Claire Plimmer for commissioning this edition. I'm also grateful to Anna Martin, Sarah Scott and Sophie Martin for their very helpful editorial input.

Contents

Author's Note

While I was writing this book, a work colleague voiced a popular misconception when she commented: 'But there's no such thing as IBS is there? Isn't it all just in the mind?' She highlighted the fact that, because IBS has been linked to psychological factors, many people don't view it as an actual health condition. My response, based on my own experiences and those of a couple of close friends, as well as my findings from researching this book, was a resounding 'Yes, there is such a thing as IBS!' I then explained that, yes, it had been linked to psychological issues, but there were very real physical symptoms, too.

Many of us will suffer from IBS at some point in our lives.

While the condition isn't life-threatening, it can make everyday life – going to work, shopping, socialising, etc. – difficult and even embarrassing. As is the case for most health conditions, there is no magic formula that will work for everyone, so I have included a wide variety of both conventional and alternative approaches in the hope that every reader will find effective ways to manage their individual IBS symptoms.

Wendy Green

Foreword

From the numerous letters and phone calls I receive from people with IBS, I recognise that Wendy Green's 50 top tips cover the issues that people with IBS need to know about: what to eat, how to deal with stress, the role of bacteria and yeasts, helpful herbs, complementary therapies and how to manage your IBS as part of your daily life. Her book finishes with a useful, comprehensive jargon buster.

Wendy's approach is holistic; she gives as much weight to herbal treatments, stress reduction and complementary therapies as to conventional drugs. She doesn't confine herself to treatments for which there is medical evidence, but instead offers a broad-based explanation of the ideas and treatments that people have found useful. This is not a book written for doctors or researchers, it is written for anyone who suffers with IBS. It recognises the personal nature of the illness and accommodates the enormous variations in symptoms and presentation. The case studies highlight this personal approach. Wendy emphasises the identification of personal IBS triggers and acknowledges that these are highly individual. Once you are aware of your triggers, you can do something about them.

Dr Nick Read,
chair of The IBS Network

I was particularly impressed by her common-sense tips to stress reduction: 'Live in the moment', 'Find social support', 'Be assertive', 'Laugh more' and 'Have a hug'. The sections on travelling without fear, helpful herbs and do-it-yourself complementary therapies are also very useful, and rarely found in other self-help books.

Wendy Green writes in a practical and accessible manner. She doesn't preach any particular therapy; she just offers people the information they need in order to find their own way. The advice in her book complements the approach adopted by The IBS Network (formerly known as The Gut Trust), the national charity for IBS, and will help many IBS sufferers to support themselves.

Introduction

Irritable Bowel Syndrome (IBS) comprises a range of conditions linked to a disturbance of the large bowel that can lead to various unexplained symptoms, including abdominal pain, bloating, diarrhoea and constipation. It affects up to one in three of the UK population at some time in their lives, but it usually first develops during teenage years and early adulthood. It is often a chronic condition, though there may be spells where the symptoms completely disappear, only to return at a later time. The symptoms can also change. While IBS is not life-threatening, it can severely disrupt daily life – for example, having to rush to the loo frequently while at work, travelling or socialising is inconvenient and embarrassing. The symptoms can range from mild to severe: some people with IBS suffer only occasional problems – perhaps only when they eat a particular food – while others experience symptoms that are so severe that they are regularly absent from work and even a simple shopping trip can be a nightmare. Up to one in five people are thought to be suffering from IBS at any one time. However, only around one in ten people will consult their GP about IBS-type symptoms – probably because most sufferers find discussing their bowel problems too embarrassing, or believe that their symptoms will eventually go away of their own accord. Two to three times as many women experience IBS symptoms as men – probably because female hormones appear to be involved. It is also more common in the Western world, which suggests that IBS, like many health problems of the twenty-first century, is linked to a stressful lifestyle, as well as an over-reliance on fatty, sugary, refined foods and a lack of exercise.

This book explains how dietary, psychological, genetic and hormonal factors may all play a part, as may suffering from gastroenteritis, bacterial imbalance and yeast infections, taking antibiotics and other drugs, and even having insufficient sleep. While there is no one cure that 'fits all', it is possible to manage your symptoms with lifestyle changes and, in some cases, appropriate medication. The key is identifying the type of IBS you are suffering from and your own particular triggers. This book provides information to help you do this, and to learn which approaches might work best for you. You will discover which dietary changes are recommended for your particular symptoms and how stress management could help you. Beneficial exercises and techniques from complementary therapies that could provide relief are also included. At the end of the book, you'll find details of useful products and books, as well as contact information for relevant organisations.

Chapter 1

About IBS

This chapter gives you an overview of the symptoms and possible causes of IBS, along with advice on preparing for a visit to your GP. The chapter ends with some IBS sufferers' stories.

The ABC of IBS

The National Institute for Clinical Excellence (NICE) recommends that anyone reporting any of these symptoms for at least six months should be assessed for IBS:

- Abdominal pain and discomfort

- Bloating

- Change in bowel habits

1 Determine whether you have IBS

The following symptoms checklist will help you decide whether or not you could have IBS.

Abdominal pain and discomfort

Abdominal pain is the main symptom of IBS. The pain is usually felt below the belly button, but can sometimes be felt all over the abdominal area. It can be a result of bloating or of the gut contracting more strongly or frequently than usual. The pain is often relieved by going to the loo.

Bloating

Another key symptom of IBS. Bloating is usually worse after a meal and in the evening. Various things can cause bloating – including pregnancy and obesity – but if you have IBS it is usually the result of a build-up of excess wind or of constipation.

Change in bowel habits

A change in bowel habits is another major sign of IBS. You may experience alternate bouts of diarrhoea or constipation.

Rumbling tummy and excessive wind

Rumbling noises coming from your stomach (borborygmi) can be embarrassing. If they're not caused by hunger, they are likely to signal excess wind. Excess wind may be caused by gulping air while eating, swallowing air when feeling anxious, drinking fizzy drinks, or abnormal fermentation of food in the gut. Studies suggest that wind passes through the gut more slowly in IBS sufferers and that they may be hypersensitive to its effects.

An urgent need to visit the loo

A common feature of IBS is needing to visit the loo urgently. This often happens while eating, or shortly afterwards, and is probably the most distressing and inconvenient aspect of the condition. This is thought to be a result of an exaggerated gastrocolic reflex – the involuntary reflex where food in the stomach stimulates activity in the bowel and results in the urge to pass a stool.

Passing mucus from your back passage

Mucus acts as a lubricant in the bowel. If you notice it in your stools, it suggests the bowel is being irritated. This is quite common with IBS.

Faecal incontinence

Faecal incontinence – where wind involuntarily escapes, along with some of the contents of your bowel – is an embarrassing and inconvenient problem faced by some IBS sufferers.

A sharp pain low down inside the bottom

The correct term for this is proctalgia fugax, and it is thought to be caused by the anal sphincter going into spasm. It may be linked to constipation and not eating enough fibre.

Feeling that a bowel movement is incomplete

This could be a result of constipation or the heightened sensitivity of your gut.

Piles (haemorrhoids)

Piles can develop as a result of suffering from IBS. They are essentially varicose veins just inside the anus – though they can sometimes protrude. They can result from, or be made worse by, the frequent straining caused by constipation, which increases the pressure on the veins. Diarrhoea can also make piles worse, because of the frequency of the bowel movements. Piles can sometimes protrude and, if they become inflamed, they can be itchy, painful and sore, and can sometimes bleed. They aren't dangerous, but if you notice blood in your stools, or after a bowel movement, you should see your GP to rule out more serious conditions.

Other, less common symptoms can include:

- Nausea, headache, dizziness and ringing in the ears
- Heartburn, burping and reduced appetite
- Feeling full very quickly when eating
- More frequent urination ('irritable bladder')
- Backache and muscular and joint pains
- Tiredness, depression and anxiety
- Shortness of breath.

The symptoms can vary in severity, but are usually worse after eating. Most sufferers experience flare-ups that last between two and four days, after which their symptoms ease, or completely disappear – often for long periods of time.

Please don't self-diagnose – if you experience any of these symptoms, remember that they could also signal other conditions, including coeliac disease, ulcerative colitis, Crohn's disease and bowel cancer, so it is essential that you get a proper diagnosis by a medical professional.

2 Visit your GP

To receive the correct diagnosis and treatment, it is important to prepare for your appointment with your GP. Note down the answers to the following questions as accurately as you can before your appointment – it's easy to forget important pieces of information when you're sitting in your GP's surgery.

- Where do you feel pain?

- How would you describe the pain – aching, nagging, stabbing, crushing, constant or intermittent?

- What helps to relieve the pain?

- What makes it worse?

- How many times daily do you have a bowel movement?

- Are your stools hard, soft or watery? (Be as specific as you can – see the Bristol Scale.)

- Do your stools contain mucus?

③ **Refer to the Bristol Stool Scale**

If you suffer from diarrhoea or constipation, you are unlikely to need anyone to tell you! However, the Bristol Stool Scale, devised as a medical aid to classify stools by Heaton and Lewis at Bristol University in 1997, could be helpful when you need to explain your symptoms as accurately as possible to a medical professional. The consistency of your stools is related to how long they spend in your colon. The longer they stay there, the more water is extracted and the drier they will be when they are expelled. There are seven types of stool, ranging from hard to pass (one and two), to ideal consistency (three and four) to difficult to control (five to seven).

For an easy-to-understand illustrated Bristol Stool Scale Chart, visit Eric, The Children's Continence Charity website: www.eric. org.uk/InformationZone/Leafletsandresources.

The different types of IBS

NICE categorises IBS according to the type of bowel motion you mainly experience:

- Alternating constipation and diarrhoea – IBS-A

- Constipation predominant – IBS-C

- Diarrhoea predominant – IBS-D

This is useful for determining which dietary and lifestyle changes and medications might help you the most.

What else could it be?

There are no tests that confirm IBS, because it's the result of a disturbance in bowel function rather than any abnormality of the bowel, which is why it's known as a 'functional disorder'. In most cases, your GP will be able to diagnose IBS simply from the symptoms you describe; however, it's good practice to carry out some basic tests to rule out other conditions. A blood sample may be taken to check for anaemia, inflammation in the body or coeliac disease. Coeliac disease is a condition where nutrients and fluids are not absorbed because of damage to the intestinal wall as a result of the immune system reacting to the proteins in cereals such as wheat, rye and barley.

A stool sample may be taken to check for the presence of blood. More complex tests, such as a colonoscopy – where a special telescopic camera is used to look inside the bowel to check for inflammation or early signs of bowel cancer – are usually only carried out if you are over 45 or have symptoms that aren't typical of IBS; for example, if, as well as IBS-like symptoms, you also experience blood in your stools, unexplained weight loss or a swelling in the stomach or back passage, or if you have a family history of bowel or ovarian cancer. Inflammation may signal ulcerative colitis or Crohn's disease. Both conditions can cause colitis (an inflamed colon) and other symptoms such as bloody diarrhoea and weight loss. Ulcerative colitis only affects the rectum and colon, whereas Crohn's disease can affect any part of the digestive system. Abdominal pain and constipation that don't respond to dietary changes or laxatives could signal rectal prolapse. This is especially common in women – particularly after childbirth when the pelvic muscles are weakened and fail to support the rectum, which then collapses, preventing faeces from being expelled. This condition can be hard to detect, because the rectum usually collapses internally. Your GP may also carry out tests to exclude other causes of abdominal pain or discomfort such as diverticular disease, chronic pancreatitis, gallstones, peptic ulcer disease, cholecystitis (inflammation of the gallbladder) and gastro-oesophageal reflux disease.

Important note

Blood in your stools, unexplained weight loss, or a swelling or lump in your stomach or back passage are never symptoms of IBS, so always see your GP as soon as possible if you experience any of these.

What causes IBS?

Because the term IBS covers a range of conditions, it follows that there is likely to be more than one cause. The symptoms are thought to be a result of the gut, or a section of it, being overactive or underactive. The gut is a long muscular tube in which food is digested, starting at the mouth and ending at the bottom and including the oesophagus, stomach and the small and large bowel – also known as the small and large intestine. Rhythmic muscle contractions in the wall of the gut move food along. If these contractions become stronger or more frequent than usual, pain and diarrhoea may result. If the contractions slow down, or become irregular, there may be constipation. (For more information about the digestive system, see chapter 2.)

It is thought that various factors may affect gut activity. Check the list below – could any of these be contributing to your IBS symptoms?

Diet and eating habits

Too much fibre – especially insoluble fibre – can lead to diarrhoea-predominant IBS in some people. Too little fibre can result in constipation-predominant IBS. Intolerances and sensitivities to particular foods and drinks may trigger symptoms, especially spicy foods, fatty foods, wheat, citrus fruits, dairy foods, nuts, coffee, cola and alcohol. Eating too quickly can lead to digestive problems such as wind and bloating.

Stress and anxiety

Stress and anxiety are often implicated in IBS. Research suggests that the brain and gut are closely related via the nervous system. Stress also causes chemical changes in the brain and gut, which are thought to affect how quickly food is pushed through the system. These changes may also alter some people's gut pain threshold. Stress hormones may also irritate the lining of the intestines, leading to 'leaky gut syndrome', where partially digested food leaks through into the bloodstream, causing an allergic reaction. Eating while feeling tense often leads to excess air being swallowed – causing bloating and pain. Some people 'over-breathe' when they're anxious, which allows air to travel down the gullet and into the stomach where it becomes trapped, causing bloating and pain. A rushed, stressful lifestyle often means that people don't take the time to go to the toilet when they need to, which can lead to the bowel becoming 'lazy' and prone to constipation.

Genetics

IBS often seems to run in families, which has raised the question of whether it is an inherited condition. Research suggests that genetics may play a part, but shared lifestyles are likely to be a bigger factor. For example, children will tend to eat the same foods as other family members, and perhaps learn to react to stress in a similar way.

Female hormones

The female hormones oestrogen and progesterone appear to be implicated in IBS: many women notice a worsening of symptoms, especially cramps and diarrhoea, just before a period, when hormone levels fall.

Gut infections

Around one in six sufferers develop symptoms after suffering from viral or bacterial gastroenteritis. It's thought that infection leaves the gut more sensitive and possibly inflamed, leading to IBS symptoms. The infection itself, or the antibiotics used to treat it, may affect the balance of 'good' and 'bad' bacteria in the gut. Some believe gut infections can damage the lining of the intestines, leading to 'leaky gut syndrome'.

Bacterial imbalance

Your gut contains a balance of 'good' and 'bad' bacteria that help break down food. When there is too much 'bad' bacteria, perhaps following an infection or a course of antibiotics, gas and bloating and other IBS symptoms can result.

Yeast infection

Infection with a yeast called *Candida albicans* has been blamed for IBS symptoms. Candida is present in everyone's gut and is normally kept under control by 'good' bacteria and a healthy immune system. Problems like IBS are thought to occur when there is an overgrowth of candida, perhaps as a result of a bacterial imbalance following a course of antibiotics, or owing to a compromised immune system following a period of stress or illness. However, many conventional medical practitioners remain sceptical of the role of candida in IBS.

Medications

Some medications can trigger IBS symptoms. These include antibiotics, non-steroidal anti-inflammatories like ibuprofen and beta blockers such as atenolol. Common side effects of ibuprofen include abdominal pain and diarrhoea.

Insufficient sleep

Research suggests that symptoms are made worse by insufficient good quality sleep. This is probably because a lack of sleep increases levels of stress hormones in the body, which in turn affects gut motility.

4 Overcome your embarrassment

Most people are embarrassed about discussing their bowel habits. Having to talk about how often you go to the loo and discuss the type of stools you pass is enough to make anyone feel ill at ease. Professor Christine Norton, a gastrointestinal nurse who sees hundreds of patients with digestive problems every year, offers some great tips to help you put things into perspective and overcome your fears on the Love Your Gut website (see Directory). She urges you to remember that you aren't the first person to have a digestive problem and that your GP or nurse won't be embarrassed. She advises being as open as you can about your symptoms and using language that you feel comfortable with, such as 'poo' and 'bottom'.

Advice from actress and IBS sufferer Cybill Shepherd

The American actress Cybill Shepherd highlighted the awkwardness many IBS sufferers feel about discussing their symptoms with their GP when she said: 'For years I have been battling recurring abdominal pain, constipation and bloating. Go ahead and laugh. We laugh because we're embarrassed. In order for us to get relief we need to talk about our symptoms and stop suffering in silence.' She revealed that her doctor dismissed her condition as 'all emotional and psychological'. Eventually she found a new doctor who took her problems seriously, diagnosed IBS and prescribed medication that relieved her symptoms.

Three IBS sufferers' stories

Some IBS sufferers may find they have one trigger, while others may identify a combination of factors that are involved in their symptoms, as these IBS sufferers' stories show.

Gail, 53

Gail first began suffering from IBS in her mid-30s. She describes her symptoms as 'awful stomach cramps followed by severe diarrhoea and a bloated feeling that lasts for a few days after an attack'. After suffering from these symptoms for a couple of years, Gail visited her GP, who diagnosed IBS. Over the years, Gail has realised that situations she finds stressful, such as 'exams or interviews, bereavement and personal problems, conflict and confrontation', trigger her symptoms. Neither over-the-counter, nor prescribed medications have helped, but she has found that a supplement containing the probiotic acidophilus eases her symptoms. She has also found that regular exercise, such as aerobics and running, help both prevent and relieve her symptoms – including the bloated feeling. She now attends aerobic classes three times a week and says: 'At the moment I have my symptoms under control.'

Joanne, 58

Joanne first experienced IBS symptoms at the age of 22. Her main symptoms are bloating, pain and diarrhoea. She has linked these with eating foods that cause excess gas – especially beans and cabbage. Eating very spicy foods causes her problems too. She says that her symptoms are made worse by stress, 'especially when I have a heavy workload, or when

I feel very tired. My IBS symptoms were at their most severe when I was going through the breakdown of my marriage.' She has since found that meditation and deep-breathing exercises help her both prevent and reduce the severity of attacks. When an attack is under way, she takes the anti-diarrhoea medication Imodium to help her gain control of her symptoms.

Peter, 45

Peter, a schoolteacher, was finding it more and more difficult to cope with the wind, bloating, pain and diarrhoea he was suffering from every day – especially while he was at work. He eventually saw his GP, who immediately arranged for tests to rule out any serious conditions before diagnosing IBS. When he discussed his symptoms with his mother, she said that she had suffered from similar digestive problems in the past and had eventually linked them to wholewheat cereals. She suggested he should try swapping his wholewheat breakfast cereal for porridge. He followed her advice and, within a few days, his symptoms disappeared.

What these three case studies also demonstrate is that, while there is no outright cure for IBS, it is possible to manage your symptoms by identifying your own particular triggers and adapting your diet and lifestyle accordingly, as well as finding supplements or medications that can help. In this book you will find information and advice on diet, supplements, stress management and relaxation techniques, as well as on over-the-counter and prescription-only medications and DIY complementary therapies that may ease symptoms.

Chapter 2

Eat to Ease IBS

This chapter provides a brief overview of how the digestive system works and suggests basic changes you can make to your eating habits that might help relieve symptoms of IBS. If these prove to be of no benefit, the next step is to look at which dietary changes might help your particular symptoms.

Many IBS sufferers are able to make a direct link between their symptoms and particular foods they eat. When the gastroenterology department at Addenbrooke's Hospital, Cambridge, conducted an audit of 500 patients with IBS in 2007, 75 per cent were deemed suitable for treatment through diet. Of these, around 65 per cent 'had a very good response' to dietary changes. This suggests that almost half of IBS sufferers can prevent, or at least greatly reduce, the number and severity of attacks through dietary changes alone. Other studies have reported similar findings.

Probably the most important aspect of dietary modification is the amount and type of fibre you eat, so different types of fibre and the part they play in IBS are evaluated below. Food intolerances appear to be implicated in some people's symptoms, so the value of keeping a food diary to help you determine whether or not they play a part in your symptoms is discussed. IBS is an individual condition, which is why foods and drinks that one person finds helpful may make things worse for another. For this reason, I have included the results of a survey that illustrate this point. Foods that commonly cause problems and the possible reasons why are identified. The role that gut bacteria play in digestion and IBS symptoms is explained and the possible benefits of probiotic supplementation are discussed. The chapter ends with advice from three well-known nutritional therapists.

How your digestive system works

To help you understand your symptoms and how dietary changes could ease them, let's take a closer look at how your digestive system works.

Digestion involves the mixing of food and drink with digestive juices, pushing them along the digestive system, and breaking them down into the smallest possible parts to enable them to be absorbed into the bloodstream through the walls of the intestines.

The digestive system (or tract) consists of the mouth, oesophagus, stomach, small intestine, large intestine (colon, or large bowel), rectum (back passage) and anus (bottom). These hollow organs are lined with a mucous membrane called mucosa. The mucosa in the mouth, stomach and small intestine has tiny glands that release juices to help digestion. Inside the digestive tract there is also a layer of smooth muscle that contracts to help break down food and push it along.

The average length of time it takes for food to pass through the digestive system is about 18 hours, depending on the speed of the muscle contractions and the content of the food. Carbohydrates take the least time to be digested. Proteins take longer and fats the longest.

Chewing your food breaks it into smaller pieces and mixes it with saliva that contains an enzyme called amylase, which begins breaking down carbohydrate into a sugar called maltose.

When you swallow food, muscle contractions (peristalsis) force it down the oesophagus to your stomach. Here it is churned and mixed with gastric juice, which contains protease, an enzyme that breaks down protein, and hydrochloric acid, which kills bacteria. The resulting thick liquid is known as chyme. The mucosa in your stomach produces mucus to protect its lining from the acid and protease, helping to lubricate the food and make it easier to push along the digestive tract.

The chyme then passes into the duodenum, the first part of your small intestine (paradoxically, the longest section of the gut), where bile is released to neutralise acids and dissolve fats in the partially digested food. This enables enzymes in the pancreatic juices to further break down carbohydrates and proteins, and begin digesting fats.

The semi-liquid then passes into the second part of the small intestine – the jejunum. The jejunum releases more of the enzymes that break down carbohydrate, proteins and fats, to turn them into glucose, amino acids and glycerol, which are then absorbed into the bloodstream.

The digested food particles then travel into the last part of the small intestine – the ileum – where vitamin B12 is absorbed and bile salts are reabsorbed. Finally, the residue travels into the large intestine, where bacteria such as *Lactobacillus acidophilus* and *Escherichia coli* help break it down (ferment it) further, producing vitamins such as biotin and vitamin K. These vitamins, and water, are absorbed in the large intestine. Undigested, insoluble fibre, bacteria, dead skin cells from the digestive tract lining, proteins, fats and water form faeces that are stored in the rectum, before being passed out through the anus.

Did you know?

Your stomach releases up to 3 litres of gastric juices a day.

Your small intestine is about 6.6 metres long.

Finger-like projections called villi increase the small intestine's surface area to the size of two tennis courts.

Your large intestine is only 1.5 metres long, but it is much wider than the small intestine.

Your large intestine contains trillions of bacteria, weighing about 1 kg in total.

What can go wrong?

If the muscle contractions in the gut are too slow, or too fast, problems can occur within the digestive process. If they're too slow, you may become constipated. If they're too fast, you may develop diarrhoea.

Constipation

Constipation, also known as 'irregularity', is a condition where the bowel movements aren't frequent enough (three bowel movements or less a week) and the faeces are hard and difficult to pass. In most people, this happens when the colon has absorbed too much water from the food passing through it. The slower the food travels along the digestive tract, the more water will be absorbed from it and the drier and harder the faeces will be. Emptying the bowels when you have constipation can be very painful. Causes of constipation include not eating enough fibre, not drinking enough fluids, not taking enough exercise, taking certain medications (such as antidepressants and certain painkillers), changes in your daily routine (for example, going on holiday), and pregnancy. As well as being a symptom of IBS, constipation is frequently the underlying cause of the condition. The difference between simple constipation and constipation-predominant IBS is that there is abdominal pain with IBS.

Diarrhoea

Diarrhoea is the passing of frequent, watery stools and can be acute or chronic. Acute diarrhoea is often caused by a viral or bacterial infection and usually clears up within a day or two. Because of the risk of dehydration, it can be serious in babies, the frail and the elderly. Chronic diarrhoea may be linked to IBS, or may be a sign of a more serious condition. It should always be investigated by your GP. Diarrhoea is generally caused by irritation of the lining of the small or large intestine, which can be a result of infection or sensitivity to a particular food, for example. The irritation can make contractions stronger and faster, which means food passes through the digestive system more quickly and there is less time for water and nutrients to be absorbed. Hence, the stools are more watery and often contain particles of undigested food. The strong contractions cause cramping pains.

5 Adopt good eating habits

Before you make any dietary changes, it is worth following these eating guidelines in order to help the digestive system operate more efficiently and to reduce the likelihood of problems like wind, bloating and diarrhoea.

- Eat at regular times – this will help your digestive system to establish a routine.

- Eat little and often – eating too much in one go can cause bloating and diarrhoea.

- Eat slowly – gulping your food down quickly can cause you to swallow air, which results in wind and bloating.

- Chew your food well to give enzymes in your saliva more time to digest it, and to stimulate gastric juices.

- Drink plenty of fluids, especially water – water combines with fibre in the intestine to make your stools bulkier and easier to pass, and it rehydrates you if you have diarrhoea.

If your symptoms persist, you may benefit from making changes to your diet. Probably the most important aspect is modification of the amount and type of fibre you eat. But first of all, let's look at how fibre fits into the picture.

Fibre and IBS

Fibre is indigestible plant matter. A diet high in fibre offers many health benefits. These include reducing the risk of constipation, piles, diverticular disease, bowel cancer, breast cancer in premenopausal women, Type 2 diabetes and coronary heart disease.

There are two types of fibre: soluble and insoluble (roughage). Most plant foods contain a combination of the two. Soluble fibre is mainly found in plant cells and insoluble fibre is found in the plant cell walls. High-fibre foods are classified according to the type of fibre that they contain the most.

Soluble fibre is mainly found in:

- Grains – including oats, barley and rye
- Vegetables – including potatoes, sweet potatoes, parsnips and carrots
- Pulses – such as beans, peas and lentils
- Fruits – such as apples, pears, bananas and strawberries.

Insoluble fibre (roughage) is mostly found in:

- Wholegrain cereals – such as wholemeal bread, wholewheat and bran cereals, and brown rice and pasta
- The skins of fruit and vegetables
- Nuts and seeds.

Both types of fibre provide bulk, which stimulates the bowel to push food through the gut, helping to prevent constipation. Fibre also absorbs water from the gut, which makes the stools bigger and softer and therefore easier to pass. As dietary fibre 'feeds' bacteria, it increases their numbers, which means that more are passed out in the faeces. This is another reason why fibre makes the faeces bulkier. For good gut health, a diet containing both types of fibre is generally recommended. The recommended daily amount is 18 g, but some studies report that 30 g or more is needed to protect gut health. If you suffer from IBS, the situation regarding your fibre intake may be more complex.

In the past, a high-fibre diet was universally recommended for IBS sufferers. However, research suggests that a high-fibre diet isn't beneficial for everyone. In 2009, researchers at the University of North Carolina School of Medicine reviewed the evidence regarding the role of diet in IBS and concluded that insoluble fibre may make symptoms worse, while an increased intake of soluble fibre improved some people's symptoms – especially those with constipation. In another survey, just over half of patients with IBS reported that fibre from cereal worsened their symptoms. Heather Van Vorous, an IBS sufferer in the US, claims that many IBS sufferers have been helped by the soluble fibre-based diet that she advocates (see Help for IBS in the Directory).

These findings are thought to be a result of the different ways in which the two types of fibre are digested. Soluble fibre, as its name suggests, dissolves in water in the gut to produce a jelly-like solution that is quickly and easily broken down (fermented) by bacteria and may soothe the gut lining. Soluble fibre also acts as a prebiotic, which means it stimulates the growth and activity of 'good' bacteria in the gut. These bacteria help in the digestion of food – their role and benefits will be discussed in more detail further on in this chapter. Examples of soluble fibre include pectin, found in apples and pears, and beta glucan, found in oats.

Insoluble fibre doesn't dissolve in water. It is only partially broken down by bacteria, so it passes through the digestive tract virtually unchanged. Its fermentation process is longer than that of soluble fibre, so more wind is produced. This causes bloating and pain in many IBS sufferers. In some people, insoluble fibre also seems to irritate the intestinal lining, which increases gut contractions and causes diarrhoea. The NICE guidelines recommend adjusting your fibre intake according to your symptoms.

6 Adjust your fibre intake

For IBS-A and IBS-D sufferers

If you have IBS-A or IBS-D, try eating less insoluble fibre and more soluble fibre, as soluble fibre is less likely to irritate the gut lining. It is also less likely to cause wind and bloating, because it is quickly broken down. Replace wholemeal bread, wholewheat cereals and wholegrain rice with foods rich in soluble fibre, such as porridge, oatcakes and oat bread. Dr Stephen Middleton, a consultant gastroenterologist at Addenbrooke's Hospital, Cambridge, noticed that many patients whose symptoms worsened with more fibre seemed to get better when they cut down on 'fibres that are likely to be fermented – like wheatbran'.

If the diarrhoea persists, your GP/dietician may suggest you try a low-fibre diet, which means eating white bread, pasta and rice rather than brown, and cornflakes rather than bran flakes, etc. You might find this odd advice if you have always eaten wholegrains on the understanding that they are better for your health; however, in time, you will probably be instructed to gradually reintroduce fibrous foods into your diet until you find the types and amounts that best suit your digestive system.

For IBS-C sufferers

If you have IBS-C, try increasing the amount of fibre in your diet. Do it gradually – a sudden, dramatic increase could lead to wind, bloating and diarrhoea. According to Dr Middleton, many people who suffer from constipation-predominant IBS symptoms often get better by simply increasing their fibre intake.

If you find that eating more fibre gives you problems with wind and bloating, try eating fewer insoluble fibre foods and more soluble fibre foods and see if there is an improvement.

If eating sufficient fibre-containing foods proves difficult, or if you need a short-term measure, you could try a bulking agent, which is a natural source of soluble fibre that isn't fermented in the gut. There are several types available, including sterculia, ispaghula, linseed and methyl cellulose (see chapters 3 and 6). Always drink plenty of water when taking a bulking agent, as this enables it to do its job properly.

The following table is a quick guide to adjusting your dietary fibre intake according to your symptoms.

Dietary Fibre Adjustment Guide

Adjustment to fibre intake	Diarrhoea (including alternating with constipation)	Constipation without wind and bloating	Constipation with wind and bloating	Wind and bloating only
Eat more foods high in both types of fibre		✓		
Eat fewer foods high in insoluble fibre	✓		✓	✓
Eat more foods high in soluble fibre	✓		✓	✓

According to Dr Middleton, about three-quarters of IBS sufferers whose symptoms are thought to be diet-related notice a marked improvement when they adjust their fibre intake. The quarter whose symptoms aren't helped in this way may need to consider whether a sensitivity to a particular food or foods is causing the problem.

Be aware of food sensitivities

Food sensitivity is complex but, in simple terms, there are two main forms: immediate and delayed.

Immediate sensitivity

In immediate food sensitivity, symptoms such as stomach pain and diarrhoea develop within an hour or two of eating the food. This is a true allergy, as it involves the immune system. Where the reaction is severe, it's known as anaphylaxis. Here, the symptoms are much more pronounced – there may be swelling of the lips, mouth and tongue. In extreme cases, there may be a sudden drop in blood pressure and loss of consciousness – anaphylactic shock – that in extreme cases can lead to death. Some researchers believe that people who react in this way to certain foods may have a leaky gut wall. This is where it becomes over-permeable, perhaps as a result of stress or irritants such as coffee, alcohol or some medications. In this state, it allows partially digested molecules of food to enter the bloodstream, where they trigger a response from the immune system. Research in Chicago suggests that people with allergic conditions like hay fever are over two-and-a-half times more likely to have IBS and those with eczema are almost four times more likely.

Always call an ambulance immediately if you suspect an anaphylactic reaction. If you experience milder symptoms of food sensitivity, consult your GP as soon as possible.

Delayed sensitivity

In delayed sensitivity, symptoms like bloating, stomach pain and diarrhoea appear within 6 to 24 hours of eating the trigger food. This isn't a true allergy, as it doesn't involve the immune response, and is more likely to be caused by intolerance, otherwise known as non-allergic hypersensitivity. This could be a result of low levels of digestive enzymes or a raised sensitivity to natural substances found in foods. Research suggests that delayed sensitivity is linked with IBS more often than immediate sensitivity or allergy. Some people may suffer from both immediate and delayed food sensitivity.

Foods that are known to trigger IBS

The foods most often implicated in immediate food sensitivity are usually proteins found in foods such as wheat, milk and peanuts. Even tiny amounts are enough to set off an allergic reaction.

The foods often linked to delayed food sensitivity are likely to be food staples, so wheat and milk are common causes in the Western world.

Common culprits include grains (especially wheat); dairy products (milk, cheese and eggs); peanuts; tree nuts (almonds, hazelnuts, pecans and walnuts); seafood, including shellfish; citrus fruits; and soy. Natural substances found in food and drink that may also be triggers include caffeine in tea and coffee; salicylates ('natural aspirin') in fruit and vegetables; and histamines in strawberries, chocolate and cheese. Sensitivity to food additives, such as sulphites and nitrates, can also be a factor. Yeasts found in bread, blue cheeses and beer have also been known to cause a reaction.

Wheat

We've already looked at the problems that the insoluble fibre (bran) contained in wholewheat can cause. Wheat also contains a common allergen: a protein called gliadin, which is found in gluten. This is why people with a wheat allergy are sometimes advised to eat a gluten-free diet. Most supermarkets now stock wheat-free breads, cakes and flours.

Dairy foods

Milk and cream contain lactose, a naturally occurring sugar that some people have problems digesting, usually because they don't produce the enzyme lactase to break it down, resulting in symptoms such as diarrhoea, constipation and cramping. However, certain dairy products, for example, yogurt, cheese and buttermilk, might not trigger IBS symptoms because the bacteria they contain breaks down the lactose.

Some full-fat dairy foods, such as Cheddar cheese or cream cheese, are high in fat, which can also be an IBS trigger, so changing to lower-fat versions may help. Additionally, the proteins in dairy – mainly casein and whey – may cause digestive problems in some people. If you're affected, you could replace cow's milk with soya milk, which is widely available. Most soya milk brands contain added calcium, which is essential for a healthy nervous system and strong bones. You could also try soya-based yogurts, cheeses and desserts.

Peanuts

Peanuts are one of the commonest causes of food allergy and many IBS sufferers believe they make their symptoms worse. They contain various allergens that aren't destroyed by cooking. In fact, roasting peanuts makes them more likely to cause an allergic reaction. Even tiny amounts of peanut can cause a reaction in individuals who are sensitive to them.

Non-citrus fruits

Non-citrus fruits may also aggravate IBS in some people. Fruit contains fructose (fruit sugar), which some people have problems digesting. In a study published in the *American Journal of Gastroenterology*, 101 out of 183 IBS sufferers experienced wind, bloating, pain and changes in their bowel movements after eating a meal high in fructose. Rather than cutting out the offending fruits altogether, try reducing the amount you eat, or eating them cooked, e.g. stewed or baked apples, as this often makes them easier to digest.

Citrus fruits

Many IBS sufferers report increased symptoms after consuming fruits like lemons, limes, oranges and grapefruits. The exact reason why these fruits cause problems is unclear, though it has been suggested it may be because of their citric acid content, as well as the fructose they contain.

Sugar and sugar substitutes

Sugar is made up of glucose and fructose. It is probably the fructose content that causes problems for some people. If you're affected, cut your intake of sweets, cakes, biscuits, desserts and chocolate and, where possible, opt for low-sugar versions of cereals and yogurts. However, be careful with foods containing sugar substitutes. Some people suffer from wind, bloating and diarrhoea when they eat sugar-free foods, sweets, mints or gum, as they contain artificial sweeteners, such as sorbitol, xylitol and mannitol, which can be difficult to digest.

Sulphites

E223 sodium metabisulphite and sulphites E221–E228 release sulphurous acid, which can irritate the lining of the stomach.

Nitrates

Nitrates such as E252 potassium nitrate, used to preserve cooked meats and sausages, can cause stomach pains in some people.

Fatty foods

Fatty foods can trigger IBS because fat stimulates the liver to release bile to break it down. Bile contains acids that can irritate a sensitive gut. Foods that can cause this kind of problem include fried foods, pastry, fatty chicken skin, full-fat cheeses, fatty meats and chocolate. If you're affected, try cutting down on these foods and taking the following steps:

- Opt for reduced-fat cheeses
- Trim all visible fat from meat
- Grill, bake, poach, steam or microwave rather than frying food
- Watch out for hidden fats in ready meals, takeaways, cakes, biscuits and pastries.

Don't cut out fats from your diet completely – your body needs them for vital bodily functions, including transporting and absorbing the fat-soluble vitamins A, D, E and K, and cushioning the vital organs. Fats are also essential for brain health, lubricating your skin and gut, and helping to make food more appetising and more filling because they slow down glucose absorption. Yet, while some fats are beneficial to health, others are detrimental.

Until recently, people were advised to avoid saturated fats. However, new research suggests that some of the saturated fats found in full-fat dairy products, such as whole milk, butter and yogurt, may boost health – they are thought to cut the risk of diabetes and heart disease, and help weight management by keeping you fuller for longer. Butter (especially grass-fed) is also a good source of vitamin A.

On the other hand, processed meats – especially sausages, bacon and burgers – should be eaten sparingly because they contain saturated fats that are linked with coronary heart disease, stroke, atherosclerosis (hardening of the arteries) and breast cancer.

Trans-fats are best avoided, too, because they're linked with hardened arteries, heart disease, diabetes and cancer. Trans-fats, also known as partially hydrogenated fats or oils, are solid fats made from vegetable oils using a process called hydrogenation. They tend to be used for frying and to increase the shelf life of shop-bought baked goods like biscuits, cakes, pastries and pies.

Opt instead for foods containing omega-3 and omega-6 fatty acids, which are anti-inflammatory. Good sources of omega-3 include oily fish, such as pilchards, sardines, salmon and mackerel, as well as dark green vegetables, nuts, seeds, egg yolks and linseed (flaxseed), hemp and rapeseed oils. Omega-6 can be found in sunflower and corn oils, olives, nuts, seeds and wholegrains.

Natural relief from constipation

Try taking 1 to 2 tablespoons of cold-pressed oil, such as olive, flaxseed, safflower or sesame oil, once a day to lubricate the digestive tract and relieve constipation.

Spicy foods

Some spices, such as chillies, are known to speed up gut contractions. It is thought that these spices irritate the gut lining. For some people with IBS, this can mean increased episodes of diarrhoea and abdominal cramping.

Vegetables

Some vegetables, such as cabbage, broccoli and onions, can cause excess gas, even in people without digestive problems. However, when these foods are eaten by people with IBS, severe bloating and cramping can sometimes result – possibly because they are more sensitive to the effects of the gas produced or because the food moves more slowly through their digestive systems.

Pulses

Pulses, such as beans, peas and lentils, can also cause excess gas, bloating and cramping in some IBS sufferers.

For further information about food intolerance, visit Allergy UK's website (see Directory).

Select Food is an online directory of companies that sell food for people with allergies, such as to wheat and dairy. For further details, see Directory.

Gut bacteria and food intolerance

Professor John Hunter, a consultant at Addenbrooke's Hospital, and other researchers have suggested that food intolerances could be a result of abnormal fermentation of food residues in the gut, caused by changes in the types and levels of bacteria found there.

What are these bacteria?

Beneficial bacteria, such as lactobacilli, bifidobacteria and *Escherichia coli*, perform an important role in digestion by helping to break food down further and making important minerals like magnesium and calcium easier to absorb. They also prevent the more harmful strains of bacteria from multiplying by using up all of the available oxygen and nutrients.

Meanwhile, the gut provides a safe environment in which these bacteria can live – making it a mutually beneficial relationship. Lactobacilli tend to live in the small intestine, while bifidobacteria are more often found in the large intestine.

Where do gut bacteria come from?

The gut of a newborn baby is sterile. During birth and breastfeeding, bacteria are transferred from mother to baby. Bacteria are also transferred from other people in the course of everyday living. These bacteria grow and multiply massively – the average adult has trillions of bacteria in the intestines, ranging over 400 different species.

Gut bacteria – the 'good' and the 'bad'

Problems arise when levels of 'good' bacteria are reduced, perhaps due to a bout of gastroenteritis or following a course of antibiotics, which destroy every type of bacteria in their wake. With fewer 'good' bacteria present, the harmful strains, known as pathogens, are able to multiply.

Research suggests that many IBS sufferers have lower levels of 'good' bacteria and higher levels of 'bad' bacteria, such as some forms of E. coli and clostridia, in the gut. These 'bad' bacteria give off excessive amounts of gases and toxic waste products when they ferment food residues in the bowel, causing wind, bloating, pain and diarrhoea. This process is known as malfermentation. Professor Hunter and other experts believe that certain foods, such as wheat and dairy products, may actually cause these changes in gut bacteria in some people.

Gut bacteria and candida yeast infection

Candida is an organism that can exist as yeast or a fungus. It can be found in dark, moist areas of the body, including the mouth, the digestive and genito-urinary tracts, and on the skin. It is thought that 'good' bacteria, bowel enzymes and immune cells control the number of yeasts in the gut, but if there aren't enough 'good' bacteria in the gut, the immune system is depleted, or if a sugary diet is eaten, candida can grow out of control and have a detrimental effect on an individual's health. Common symptoms include thrush, and some people believe irritable bowel syndrome can also be caused by candida overgrowth. It is claimed that it is the chemicals produced by candida – alcohol and acetaldehyde – that cause health problems.

Another theory is that candida can sometimes switch from its yeast form into a fungus that grows 'branches' that can penetrate the wall of the gut, causing 'leaky gut syndrome'. 'Leaky gut syndrome' is a condition proposed by some health practitioners in which particles of undigested food pass through the gut walls into the bloodstream where they provoke an immune response. However, the medical profession is generally sceptical of these claims.

If candida is suspected, probiotics to restore 'good' bacteria, and a low-yeast and low-sugar diet, are recommended. This means avoiding yeast-containing foods and drinks, such as bread, beer, wine, vinegar, pickles, mushrooms, black olives, peanuts and vitamin B supplements, unless 'yeast-free' is written on the label. Refined carbohydrates, including sugar, should also be avoided, as they encourage the growth of candida in the body. If you want to learn more about the theories that link candida to IBS, The Henry Spink Foundation's website offers more detailed information. Contact details are in the Directory section.

8 Boost your beneficial bacteria

Research suggests that boosting the levels of 'good' bacteria in your gut may help control your IBS symptoms. Five randomised placebo-controlled trials demonstrated that probiotics are especially good for reducing wind and bloating. According to the World Health Organization (WHO), probiotics are 'live micro-organisms which, when administered in adequate amounts, confer a health benefit on the host'.

For foods to be described as probiotic, the WHO says they must have these properties:

- A sufficient number of 'good' bacteria that remain alive and active until the end of the shelf-life of the product.

- Bacteria that must be able to survive strong stomach acids.

- Identified probiotic bacteria, whose specific type and strain is named.

Probiotics from the *Lactobacillus* and *Bifidobacterium* families, and a strain called *Streptococcus thermophilus*, seem to be the most beneficial. There are probiotic yogurt drinks on the market, such as Yakult and Actimel, both of which contain strains of *Lactobacillus*. Actimel also contains *Streptococcus thermophilus*. Some drinks can be high in sugar and may contain fructose, so choose the light versions where possible. You can also buy probiotic supplements, although some of these can be expensive. See chapter 3 and the Useful Products section for further information.

Natural and fruit bio-yogurts can be used as alternatives, but the drinks and supplements tend to offer the highest doses of probiotics – usually at least ten million live bacteria per dose – which means that more are likely to survive the acids in the stomach. You will probably need to take probiotics every day for at least a month before you notice any benefits.

Some probiotic supplements have prebiotics added – these are natural sugars that feed 'good' bacteria and encourage them to multiply. They are usually listed as either insulin (found in vegetables) or fructo-oligosaccharides (FOS), which are found in fruit. Prebiotics seem to benefit those who suffer from IBS-C the most. If you have IBS-D, treat such supplements with caution as some research suggests that prebiotics can make diarrhoea or bloating worse. Foods rich in prebiotics include artichokes, leeks, celery, cucumber and tomatoes.

9 Keep a food diary

Different foods affect individuals in different ways – what triggers IBS symptoms in one person may relieve them in another, so it makes sense to track your symptoms and current diet before making any changes. The best way to do this is to keep a food and symptom diary; an ordinary notebook will do. For two weeks, write down everything you eat each day and any symptoms that follow. Make sure you remember to include snacks and drinks, and list all of the ingredients in a meal. For example, if you eat a curry, record all of the spices used to help you identify which one, if any, is causing problems. It might also be worth noting other aspects of the meal. Were you in such a hurry that you gulped your food down? Were you feeling anxious about something while you were eating?

After two weeks, examine your diary entries. If you notice a pattern emerging that suggests that a particular food or foods seem to trigger your IBS symptoms, the next step should be to visit your GP armed with this information.

It's not a good idea to attempt to exclude a major food group without guidance from your GP or a dietician. For example, if you conclude that dairy foods are at the root of your problems, cutting them out could leave you short of calcium, which is vital for a healthy nervous system, bones and teeth. A dietician might suggest alternatives, such as tinned sardines, dark green leafy vegetables, almonds, calcium-fortified soya products, or even a calcium supplement. You may notice that your symptoms are linked to the way you eat, rather than what you eat. If you rush your food or eat while feeling anxious, you might be swallowing too much air, resulting in uncomfortable wind and bloating.

🔟 Try an exclusion diet

An exclusion diet is sometimes recommended to help determine whether your symptoms are linked to a particular food or foods. A basic exclusion diet involves simply eliminating a food you suspect brings on your symptoms from your diet. A multiple exclusion diet, as the name suggests, involves cutting out more than one suspected food. A restriction diet is far more extreme and involves eating only a few foods. For example, the Addenbrooke's Hospital's exclusion diet allows only chicken, turkey, lamb, pork, liver and kidney, fresh and tinned fish and shellfish, non-citrus fruit and rice (ground, boiled, cakes, etc.). It doesn't allow wheat, oats, rye, corn or barley, dairy foods, tea, coffee, alcohol or fizzy drinks, chocolate, sweets, nuts, or foods containing yeast. The omitted foods are then gradually reintroduced.

It's important to keep a food and symptom diary, both during the food exclusion and the food reintroduction periods. If you react to a particular food, remove it from your diet again. Eventually, after a process of trial and error, you will learn which foods are responsible for your symptoms. According to Professor Hunter, food intolerances can change – you might find you can eat foods again that once caused you problems, although perhaps only in small amounts. Therefore, he advises rechecking what you are intolerant to every six months.

Changing your diet needn't be a problem – most supermarkets now stock wheat-free and dairy-free products, including flours, milks and spreads, enabling you to adapt your favourite recipes. See the Recipe section at the end of the book for examples of wheat- and dairy-free dishes.

The low-FODMAP diet

This is a type of elimination diet developed in Australia, in 1999, by nutritionist Dr Sue Shepherd and gastroenterologist Dr Peter Gibson, and is now widely accepted as an effective treatment for many IBS sufferers. FODMAP stands for fermentable oligosaccharides, disaccharides, monosaccharides and polyols. These are all types of sugars that some people have problems digesting. High-FODMAP foods include many of those we've already discussed, such as wheat, dairy, sugar and sugar substitutes, and certain fruits and vegetables, including apples, onions and cabbage.

Please note

Any exclusion diet should only be undertaken under the supervision of a dietician or other suitably qualified medical professional, as they can be difficult to follow on your own and nutritional deficiencies can result from cutting out whole food groups. There are trained low-FODMAP dietitians working in the NHS and privately. If you want to see an NHS dietitian, you can ask your GP or consultant to refer you. For more information about the diet, see the Helpful Books section and the Directory.

Exclusion diet: a case study

Carol Sinclair's story

Carol Sinclair had suffered from IBS symptoms since childhood. Her symptoms had worsened during her teenage years and, by middle age, severe bloating and pain were a regular occurrence. She suffered constantly from constipation and was advised to increase her fibre intake. She had always eaten high-fibre foods, like brown bread and bran muffins, but she began to eat more of these foods. However, she still had bloating and pain, and her constipation got worse. She resorted to increasing her use of laxatives and went on to try yogurt and various herbs and other remedies, but without success.

Then, in 1986, she watched a documentary featuring Professor John Hunter's research on food allergies and IBS that suggested that giving up wheat could eliminate IBS symptoms. She immediately cut wheat flour, wholegrains and wheat bran from her diet, and found that her symptoms decreased dramatically. After about a year and a half, she began experiencing her symptoms again, intermittently. She was admitted to St Mark's Hospital in London for tests to find out if she had a condition called Hirschsprung's disease, where part of the bowel is paralysed. The tests proved inconclusive. During her stay, she was encouraged to swap the laxatives, to which she had unknowingly become addicted, for Epsom salts. She says that this advice alone made the two weeks she spent undergoing uncomfortable tests worthwhile.

Carol spent the next few years trying to discover which foods – apart from wheat – were causing her symptoms, and concluded that it was starch. Since completely excluding starches from her diet she has been symptom-free. She believes that the type of IBS she suffers from is one of a number of inflammatory diseases, which include a form of arthritis called ankylosing spondylitis (AS) and can be identified by a specific genetic marker. Professor Alan Ebringer, an immunologist at King's College, London, says that eating lots of dietary starch encourages the growth of a bacteria called klebsiella in the gut, which he believes triggers AS and IBS in genetically susceptible people. Information on Carol's book *The IBS Low-Starch Diet: Why starchy food may be hazardous to your health*, in which she outlines her experiences and details the low-starch diet that brought her relief, can be found in the Helpful Books section.

IBS sufferers' dietary survey

In 2005, the IBS Research Appeal conducted a survey of IBS sufferers – 98 per cent of whom had been diagnosed by a medical professional – on foods and drinks they avoided and those they believed helped them. There were 400 participants (322 women aged 18–91 and 78 men aged 25–82) and their symptoms ranged from occurring every day to just once a year. The study showed quite clearly that foods and drinks that aggravated symptoms in one person eased them in another: quite literally, 'One man's meat is another man's poison.' These diverse results are probably caused by individual food sensitivities and whether symptoms are constipation- or diarrhoea-predominant.

This wasn't a clinical trial; it was based on the participants' own perceptions, but the results back up clinical findings that have consistently found dairy foods – wheat products; vegetables, such as cabbage, beans, broccoli and onions; citrus fruits; sugar and sugar substitutes, such as sorbitol; and spicy foods – to be most commonly linked to IBS. Research shows that the drinks most commonly associated with IBS are those containing caffeine, such as coffee, cola and tea; alcohol; and milk.

The researchers highlighted the fact that coffee was by far the most common drink perceived to cause digestive problems. This is probably because the caffeine in coffee stimulates gut contractions. They also noted that water, especially bottled, was by far the most popular drink for easing symptoms of IBS. Aloe vera and cranberry juices were also highly rated.

General dietary advice for IBS

What all of this shows is that there isn't one ideal diet for IBS – it really is a case of finding out for yourself which foods seem to cause your symptoms and then to avoid eating them. However, in general, a balanced diet that focuses on plain foods, and is low in trans-fats and saturated fats found in processed meats, sugar and highly spiced foods, is likely to benefit sufferers of all types of IBS. Indeed, such a diet is recommended for good health and a healthy weight.

Remember, too, that it's not just what you eat, but how you eat it. If you rush your food, you are more likely to gulp down lots of air, which can cause bloating and pain. You probably won't chew your food thoroughly enough either, which means it may not be digested properly, and if you eat while feeling tense and anxious, your digestive system may not function efficiently. For more about the relationship between your brain and your gut, see chapter 4.

⑪ Consider nutritional therapists' advice

Nutritional therapists believe that health problems such as IBS can be both prevented and treated with appropriate nutrition.

Ian Marber, one of the founders of The Food Doctor, says it's hard to make and stick to big changes in your diet, and suggests some basic dietary changes to improve your digestion. He recommends eating a tablespoon of sauerkraut daily, as it contains healthy bacteria. He believes that fruit can lead to bloating, especially when eaten directly after a main meal, and claims it's best eaten either half an hour before, or 2 hours afterwards. Marber says that eating pineapple and papaya aids digestion, because they contain the protein-digesting enzymes bromelain and papain. To boost beneficial bacteria, he advises swapping fruit yogurts for natural bio-yogurt, and warns that many probiotic drinks are high in sugar, which can cause bloating. He also recommends adding ginger, peppermint and fennel to meals, or drinking them as herbal teas, to reduce wind (see chapter 3). For more information, visit www.thefooddoctor.com.

Dr Andrew Weil, an expert in integrated medicine, claims that many people note an improvement in their IBS symptoms when they avoid dairy foods. For more details, go to www.drweil.com.

Nutritional consultant Patrick Holford agrees: he believes that most adults have an intolerance to milk, because they no longer produce the digestive enzyme lactase. Holford also recommends taking FOS (fruit sugars), which act as a prebiotic, as well as soaked oats and flaxseeds (linseed), for constipation (see chapter 3). For more details, visit www.patrickholford.com.

Nutritional therapy isn't currently available on the NHS. If you would like to consult a nutritional therapist in your area, the British Association for Applied Nutrition and Nutritional Therapy provides an online directory of qualified practitioners at bant.org.uk.

Following a restricted diet can lead to nutritional deficiencies. Always seek dietary advice from your GP if you suspect that a particular food group is causing or aggravating your symptoms.

Warning

Improve your digestion the Viva Mayr way

Dr Harald Stossier, medical director at the Viva Mayr clinic, an Austrian spa hospital popular with the rich and famous, has developed an eating programme aimed at improving digestion and banishing bloating. The programme is based on an eating plan originally created by Dr Franz Mayr over 80 years ago, as a cure for poor digestion. Although it is also designed to help weight loss, it offers sound dietary advice that some IBS sufferers may find helpful. The main guidelines are:

- Drink at least 2 litres of water every day between meals, up to 15 minutes before eating and from one hour afterwards.

- Avoid drinking water while eating, as it dilutes the enzymes in your saliva that begin the digestive process. Sipping a small glass of wine is 'allowed', as it helps to break down fats.

- Coffee and tea should be avoided because they contain caffeine, which can irritate the gut.

- Also avoid fizzy drinks, because they cause wind and bloating.

- Don't eat when stressed, or while you're on the move.

- Eat foods that are harder to digest, such as raw fruit and vegetables, before 4 p.m., because the digestive system is at its most efficient then.

- Your breakfast and lunch should be your biggest meals and your evening meal should be the smallest.

- Choose easily digestible foods in the evening, such as lightly cooked vegetables and fish, preferably no later than 6 p.m., as this is when the digestive system is beginning to slow down.

- It's better not to eat at all than to eat in a hurry, as this leads to fermentation in the gut. Chewing your food between 30 and 40 times before swallowing aids nutrient absorption.

- Base your meals on fruit and vegetables, with small amounts of good-quality proteins and fats.

- Don't overdo animal proteins: pulses, nuts and seeds provide protein in a more easily digested form. White meats such as chicken and turkey are easier to digest than red meats. Goats' and sheep's cheeses are more digestible than cheeses made from cows' milk.

- Cut down on carbohydrates, especially refined white foods. Aim to eat small portions of wholegrains, such as wholemeal bread, brown rice and wholewheat pasta.

- Two-thirds of your diet should be alkaline foods, e.g. vegetables, potatoes, ripe fruit, nuts and seeds, milk and cream, herbs, spices, and cold-pressed oils.

- Acidic foods such as meat, fish, cheese, animal fats, grains, pulses, citrus fruits, refined and processed foods, alcohol, coffee and tea should make up the remaining third of the diet.

Quick summary of dietary advice

- Eat little and often.
- Eat slowly, chewing food well.
- Drink plenty of water.
- Adjust your fibre intake according to your symptoms.
- Identify food triggers and intolerances. Limit or avoid culprits.
- Try probiotics to boost beneficial bacteria.
- Consider nutritional therapists' advice.

Chapter 3

Helpful Herbs and Soothing Supplements

This chapter looks at the various herbs, spices and supplements that have been found to ease IBS symptoms. Herbal remedies have been used for centuries in every culture around the world. However, in the Western world over the past few decades, conventional medicine has replaced herbal treatments. Many view herbal treatments with scepticism, yet many important drugs have been developed from plants. For example, aspirin comes from the willow tree and the heart drug digitoxin comes from the foxglove plant. A number of the herbs and spices that have traditionally been used for the treatment of digestive problems can be found in your kitchen cupboards or growing in your garden.

12 Try remedies from the kitchen cupboard

Before you go out and buy supplements, it may be worth trying some of these traditional remedies from your kitchen cupboard.

Handy tip

Use a cafetière to make your herbal teas quickly and easily. Put the herbs in and add boiling water. Replace the cafetière lid. Leave to brew, then press down the plunger and pour.

Aniseed

Aniseed, the liquorice-flavoured seed of the anise plant, a member of the carrot family, is used in Ayurvedic medicine as a carminative – which means it can both prevent the formation of wind and ease its passing. Herbalists have traditionally used it to relieve griping pains and aid digestion. It is thought to regulate the digestive system, making it useful for all types of IBS, and also has calming, sedative properties. The active constituent is trans-anethole, which is responsible for the distinctive taste and smell of aniseed. The seeds can be chewed or made into a tea. To make aniseed tea, lightly crush the seeds first before pouring boiling water over them. Leave to brew for about 5 minutes. Strain and drink.

Apple cider vinegar

A teaspoonful of apple cider vinegar in a glass of water before eating is a traditional remedy for digestive problems. Apple cider vinegar is made from freshly pressed apple juice that is allowed to ferment at room temperature for four to six weeks. In 1958, an American doctor called D. C. Jarvis wrote a book, *Folk Medicine: A vermont doctor's guide to good health*, about the medicinal properties of apple cider vinegar. According to Jarvis, apple cider vinegar can destroy harmful bacteria in the gut. The acetic acid and enzymes in it are thought to aid food digestion and the absorption of minerals such as calcium. The pectin from the apples may help constipation. Add a little honey to sweeten if needed, or choose a product with honey already added.

Black pepper

Black pepper has traditionally been used in Ayurvedic medicine to treat stomach disorders. Indian research suggests that using black pepper to flavour your meals will aid digestion and reduce bloating. The active ingredient appears to be piperine, which is thought to stimulate the release of hydrochloric acid via the taste buds. Try using whole black peppercorns in a grinder to enjoy the most flavour.

Caraway seeds

The ancient Greek physician Dioscorides recommended the use of caraway seeds to aid digestion. They are thought to stimulate the production of gastric juices and contain a natural antibiotic. Research suggests that the volatile oils and other chemicals in caraway help relax muscle spasms in the intestines and release trapped wind. You can make a tea by adding one cup of boiling water to 1 teaspoon of caraway seeds. Leave to infuse for about 10 minutes, strain and drink.

Cardamom

The cardamom plant is native to South East Asia, Sri Lanka and southern India and is often used in Indian cookery. Cardamom features in Ayurvedic and Chinese medicine as an anti-flatulent and an aid to indigestion. It is thought to relieve wind by easing spasms in the intestines and promoting the digestion of fats by stimulating the production of bile. The whole pods can be chewed, or try adding them to plain rice before boiling.

Camomile

Camomile is a member of the aster family. Research suggests that camomile can ease cramps and bloating by calming the muscles in the gastrointestinal tract. It is also a calming, relaxing herb, making it very useful for treating stress-related IBS. The active ingredient is the amino acid glycine, a muscle and nerve relaxant. Camomile teabags are widely available in supermarkets. Alternatively, you can grow camomile in your garden and make your own tea from the fresh or dried flower heads.

Camomile is generally safe, though you should avoid taking it if you have an allergy to the *Asteraceae* (*Compositae*) family of plants, which includes aster, chrysanthemum, mugwort, ragweed and ragwort.

Coriander

Coriander was grown as a medicinal herb by the ancient Egyptians, Chinese, Indians and Greeks, and was introduced to Britain by the Romans. Both Ayurvedic and Chinese medicine use coriander for indigestion. Some nutritional therapists recommend it for the relief of trapped wind and tummy cramps. Add the chopped leaves to curries and other savoury dishes after cooking, or add boiling water to a few fresh leaves and brew for 5 minutes before drinking.

Dill seeds

Dill seeds have traditionally been the main ingredient of gripe water to relieve colic in babies by dispersing wind and easing pain. The active constituents include volatile oils and flavonoids.

You can easily grow your own plants from the seed, either outdoors or indoors. To harvest the seeds, they must be dried by hanging the seed heads upside down in a paper bag for a couple of weeks. Once they are dry, the seeds will fall into the bag, ready for you to store them in an airtight jar.

To make dill seed tea, leave 1 to 2 teaspoons of dried seeds in a cup of boiling water for about 10 minutes, then strain and drink.

Fennel

Both the plant and the seeds have traditionally been used to ease stomach cramps and wind. Terpenoids, which have a carminative (wind-relieving) effect, are thought to be the active ingredients. Fennel is also said to stimulate the production of bile, which means it may help break down fats in food. In *The Complete German Commission E Monographs* – a guide written by the German E Commission that reviews herbal drugs and preparations from medicinal plants for their quality, safety and effectiveness – the recommended dose is 1 to 1.5 teaspoons of seeds a day.

The seeds have an aniseed flavour and are quite pleasant to chew or, if you prefer, you can make a tea using 1 teaspoon per cup of boiling water. Leave to brew for 10 to 15 minutes, then strain and drink. The plant can be eaten raw, finely sliced in salads, or roasted in a little olive oil and served with fish or chicken.

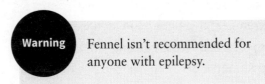

Warning Fennel isn't recommended for anyone with epilepsy.

Ginger

Ginger root has been used in traditional Ayurvedic, Chinese and herbal medicine for centuries. As well as easing nausea, ginger is thought to stimulate digestion and tone the muscles in the digestive tract to help food pass through the system more easily, causing less irritation to the intestinal walls. Ginger also contains zingibain, a digestive enzyme that helps the body break down food and aids the absorption of nutrients.

It's relatively cheap and widely available, and can be added to savoury dishes such as stir-fries and curries. You can make ginger tea by grating a 2.5-cm cube into a cup and adding boiling water. Leave to brew for 5 minutes, then strain and sweeten with honey to taste, if desired. You can also take ginger in capsule form. The recommended daily dose is usually 50–150 mg.

Peppermint

Peppermint was used by the ancient Greeks for digestive problems. Its main active ingredients (menthol, menthone and eucalyptol) are thought to ease spasms by relaxing the intestinal muscles. In 2008, the *British Medical Journal* (BMJ) reported that nearly 50 per cent of IBS sufferers found relief from their symptoms when they took peppermint oil.

You can take peppermint in tea, oil, herb or capsule form. Peppermint teabags are readily available in supermarkets, or you can add a few drops of peppermint oil to half a tumbler of warm water. You can grow your own mint in the garden or on a windowsill and use it to make a tea. Simply pour boiling water over 30 g (2 tablespoons) of the fresh herb and leave to brew for 5 to 10 minutes. Then strain and serve.

Some people claim that enteric-coated capsules work the best because they protect the active ingredients from stomach acids and are absorbed in the intestines, where they are most needed – see chapter 6 for further details.

13 Take supplements

Supplements are often controversial, with some reports claiming that isolated substances don't provide the same benefits that nutrients found in foods do. However, for many of us, supplements represent a convenient means of improving our diets or including beneficial herbs, vitamins or minerals. Often there is anecdotal evidence, but there is no, or insufficient, conclusive evidence that a supplement works. This doesn't necessarily mean that it's ineffective – often it's just that the research hasn't been done, while sometimes the type of research undertaken gives results that are deemed inconclusive. For example, if a study is carried out on only one group of participants, without a comparison group to take a different treatment or not have any treatment at all, the results may be unreliable. Or, the participant might feel an improvement because they expect to, rather than because of the treatment itself, which is known as the placebo effect.

Herbal products are most often sold as either traditional herbal registration (THR) remedies or herbal food supplements. THR products are regulated and monitored by the government agency known as the Medicines and Healthcare Products Regulatory Authority. If a product has a THR stamp it means the MHRA is satisfied it meets quality standards, has appropriate labelling and a product information leaflet. It also indicates that the herb has been used in traditional remedies for over 30 years. All THR products have a nine-digit registration number starting with the letters THR on the container or packaging.

Herbal food supplements come under the remit of the Food Standards Agency (FSA) and the Chartered Trading Standards Institute at local authority level and are not under the same legal and manufacturing scrutiny. This means there is no guarantee of their content or quality. In 2015 the School of Pharmacy at University College London tested over 70 of the herbal remedies most often bought from the high street or online and found that while most contained high amounts of the main ingredient, worryingly up to a third had very little or none at all. So it is probably best to choose THR remedies or, if a product isn't registered, check that it is from a reputable company.

Also, a few herbal medicines in the UK have a product licence. Licensed herbal medicines, like any other medicine, are required to demonstrate safety, quality and effectiveness, and to provide guidelines on safe use, so only herbal medicines with medicinal claims supported by acceptable clinical data are given product licences. They can be identified by a nine-digit number, prefixed by the letters PL.

The Department of Health's Medicines and Healthcare products Regulatory Agency (MHRA) provides a full list of herbal products currently registered under the Traditional Herbal Medicines Registration Scheme, along with information sheets on their safe use. Details can be found in the Directory at the end of this book.

Activated charcoal

Charcoal is an old-fashioned remedy for treating excess stomach and intestinal wind. The charcoal absorbs the excess gas in the gut. You can buy J. L. Bragg's Medicinal Charcoal in tablet or capsule form from health food shops, pharmacies and online (see Useful Products). Charcoal is safe to take during pregnancy and breastfeeding.

Artichoke

Artichoke is one of the oldest cultivated plants in the world – the ancient Greeks and the Romans used it as an aid to digestion. Its active constituents include cynarin, flavonoids and caffeoylquinic acids, which are thought to stimulate the production of bile. In one uncontrolled study, where 553 people with non-specific digestive disorders took 320–640 mg of a standardised artichoke extract three times a day, 70 per cent reported a reduction in abdominal pain, wind, nausea and constipation.

In recent years, artichoke has been widely used across Europe to ease digestive complaints – especially after eating fatty foods.

Calcium

Some IBS sufferers find that taking a calcium supplement helps to counteract diarrhoea. This is thought to be a result of calcium slowing down gut contractions.

Calcium is needed for strong bones and teeth, and a healthy nervous system. If you are avoiding dairy foods because you believe they are causing your IBS symptoms, it's important to ensure you eat other calcium-rich foods, such as green leafy vegetables, almonds and tinned sardines with the bones left in. If you are concerned about your calcium intake, you could try a calcium supplement. Avoid supplements containing calcium carbonate, as they may increase your chances of developing kidney stones. Instead, choose one containing calcium citrate, which is more easily absorbed, such as Solgar Calcium Citrate with Vitamin D (see Useful Products). The recommended daily intake of calcium is 800–1,000 mg.

Digestive enzymes

Taking the time to chew your food properly is probably the best way to improve your digestion. Another way is to take a digestive enzyme supplement (see Useful Products). These usually contain a combination of:

Amylase – for the digestion of carbohydrates
Betaine hydrochloric acid – to aid digestion in the stomach
Lipase – to digest fats
Papaya and bromelain (from pineapples) – for protein digestion
Pepsin and peptidase – for the digestion of protein.

Evening primrose oil

Evening primrose oil is rich in omega-6 oils and has anti-inflammatory properties. Anecdotal evidence suggests that it can even help premenstrual IBS symptoms (see chapter 5). Few adverse effects have been reported, although there have been rare cases of evening primrose oil causing seizures in people with epilepsy. The recommended daily dose is 2–4 g.

Ispaghula husks

Ispaghula husks, also known as psyllium or psyllium seed husks, come from the seeds of the plant *Plantago ovata* and have traditionally been used to treat constipation in Asia, Europe and North America. Ispaghula husks are usually taken in powder form with water. The usual dose is about 3.5 g twice a day. They are also available in their natural state, or in capsule or dried form. They soak up water to form a jelly-like mass which makes the stools bulky and soft and encourages gut contractions – provided they are taken with sufficient water. Their ability to mop up excess fluid means they are effective for diarrhoea, too. However, they may cause wind and bloating in some people. You can buy ispaghula husk supplements at most health food shops. They're also available over the counter in pharmacies as Regulan, Fybogel, and Isogel – not to be confused with High5 IsoGel, a carbohydrate energy gel – (see chapter 6).

Linseed

The German Commission E recommends linseed (also known as flaxseed) for chronic constipation and IBS. Linseed contains both soluble and insoluble fibres. The soluble fibre is contained in the mucilage – a jelly-like substance found in some plants that is thought to soothe the digestive tract by coating it with a lining. Linseed also contains omega-3 and omega-6 essential fatty acids that may have an anti-inflammatory effect on the bowel. You can buy whole linseeds or ground linseed, known as linseed meal. The recommended daily dose is 2 to 3 tablespoons of seeds or meal daily. Try mixing linseed meal with porridge oats before cooking. You can sprinkle whole linseeds over salads and bread dough to add crunch and flavour. It's important to drink plenty of water when taking linseed.

Magnesium

Magnesium is needed to aid the absorption of calcium. Most reputable calcium supplements contain magnesium at a ratio of around 2:1. Magnesium works in the opposite way to calcium by speeding up gut contractions to relieve constipation. If you have IBS-C, try taking magnesium oxide or magnesium citrate tablets. Or, you could take Epsom salts (magnesium sulphate). You may need to experiment with the amount until you find a dose that suits you.

The long-term use of laxatives is not recommended as it can lead to the bowel becoming dependent on them. Always see your GP if lifestyle changes, such as increased fibre, water and exercise, do not relieve your constipation.

Probiotics

Probiotic supplements are a convenient way of ensuring you boost your intake of 'good' bacteria, especially if you're not keen on bio-yogurt or probiotic drinks. Some experts believe that taking a high-strength probiotic supplement is the best way of ensuring that sufficient numbers of beneficial bacteria reach the intestines, because stomach acids can destroy up to half of those ingested. Professor Glenn Gibson, a microbial researcher at Reading University, recommends taking a supplement containing *Lactobacillus* and *Bifidobacterium* with at least ten million bacteria per dose. Research suggests that you need to take them every day to notice any benefit.

Slippery elm

Slippery elm supplements contain the powdered inner bark of the North American red elm tree. The active constituent is mucilage, which is thought to help calm diarrhoea. According to the botanist Dr David Bellamy, slippery elm is a 'tried and tested Aboriginal remedy' and is used in Ayurvedic medicine as a tonic. However, there is only anecdotal evidence regarding its use for IBS. Slippery elm is usually taken as a powder, which can be stirred into drinks, or taken in capsule form.

Turmeric

Various studies suggest that turmeric can help ease digestive problems. It is thought to have anti-inflammatory properties and to block abnormal muscle contractions in the gut. A small study at Reading University involving 207 IBS sufferers suggested that it can reduce abdominal pain and the frequency of diarrhoea attacks. The lead researcher, Dr Rafe Bundy, concluded that turmeric extracts can play a role in improving IBS symptoms. The recommended dosage is 500 mg of standardised turmeric extract once a day until your symptoms improve.

Chapter 4

Stress and IBS

There is a lot of evidence that psychological factors play an important role in IBS. This isn't to suggest that IBS is 'all in the mind', because the symptoms that sufferers experience are without a doubt real. However, many sufferers notice that changes in their emotional state, such as stress, anxiety or depression, are often linked to flare-ups, and research has shown that IBS is more common in people who have had a traumatic experience in the past.

A study in Chicago suggested that people suffering from depression were around two-and-a-half times more likely to suffer from IBS. In another study involving 620 people with gastroenteritis, researchers at the University of Southampton reported that those who were anxious about their symptoms, or who pushed themselves too hard and refused to rest and recuperate, were more likely to develop IBS.

This chapter looks at the various theories linking emotional stress to IBS attacks and how the symptoms themselves can cause anxiety and depression, leading to a vicious circle of emotional and physical symptoms. Stress management and relaxation techniques are suggested to both help prevent attacks and relieve tension during attacks. Hypnotherapy is another option that seems to help some IBS sufferers. For more details, see chapter 8.

> The sitcom actress Wendy Craig revealed that she suffers from stress-related IBS: 'When I'm in some kind of torment, I get indigestion and irritable bowel syndrome. I relax by listening to music.'

What is stress?

Stress is basically the way the mind and body respond to situations and pressures that leave us feeling inadequate or unable to cope. One person may cope well in a situation that another might find stressful: it's all down to the individual's perception of it and their ability to deal with it.

The brain reacts to stress by temporarily changing the body's functioning to provide the extra strength and speed needed to either stay put and fight the perceived threat or to run away from it.

It does this by releasing hormones (chemical messengers) including adrenaline, noradrenaline and cortisol into the bloodstream. These speed up the heart rate and boost levels of glucose and fats in the blood to provide a burst of energy to deal with the threat. This is called the 'fight or flight' response.

Nowadays, the situations that induce the stress response are unlikely to necessitate either of these reactions. Those pressures that continue for a long period of time with no end in sight, for example, long-term unemployment, illness or an unhappy relationship, mean that stress-hormone levels remain high, thereby increasing the risk of major health conditions such as coronary heart disease, as well as other psychological and physical symptoms. These include irritability, poor concentration, anxiety, depression, headaches, skin problems and digestive problems, such as IBS, so it's important to find ways to reduce and deal with stress.

There are various theories that link stress to IBS symptoms:

The brain–gut axis

In recent years, researchers have learned that the gut has more nerve cells than the spinal cord, and these form the enteric nervous system, which allows the brain and gut to constantly exchange messages. This means that whatever affects the brain is likely to affect the gut, and vice versa. This explains why a shock, such as bereavement or worry, can cause some people to lose their appetite. Scientists devised the term 'brain–gut axis' to describe this close relationship between the brain and the gut. This suggests that when people with IBS take steps to reduce stress, anxiety and depression by calming their mind, they can literally calm their gut as well.

Stress hormones and gut pain

When you are stressed, your body, as well as releasing adrenaline, releases a hormone called CRF (corticotropin-releasing factor), which stimulates the release of cortisol. It's thought that during prolonged stress, adrenaline and CRF affect the nerve cells in the gut, making them more sensitive to pain, so that even normal contractions are extremely painful. This could explain the abdominal pain many IBS sufferers experience when they are stressed.

Stress and 'leaky gut syndrome'

Other researchers believe that prolonged exposure to stress hormones irritates the gut lining, making it hypersensitive and prone to 'leaky gut syndrome'. This is where the gut wall becomes weakened and allows partially digested food to leak through into the blood stream, where it causes an immune response (see chapter 2).

Serotonin and IBS

Another theory is that when you are feeling stressed or depressed, there are chemical changes in your brain that affect the speed of gut contractions. Serotonin is a key brain chemical linked to mood and, interestingly, it is also released by cells in the gut walls to stimulate the contractions that push food through the digestive tract (this process is known as peristalsis). When too much serotonin is released, the gut contractions speed up, leading to diarrhoea. When too little serotonin is secreted, the gut contractions become too slow and constipation results. Antidepressant drugs called selective serotonin reuptake inhibitors (e.g. Prozac, Zoloft and Seroxat) boost mood by increasing levels of serotonin. They do this by blocking the reuptake of serotonin in the brain cells. People with constipation-predominant IBS sometimes find these antidepressant drugs helpful (see chapter

6). However, it is worth ensuring that your diet contains enough serotonin-producing foods before trying medications with potential side effects (see action 26: Sleep well on pp.92–95).

Anxiety and air swallowing

The gastroenterologist Professor John Hunter believes that some people's IBS symptoms are caused by them gulping down more air than usual when they are feeling anxious. Normal, relaxed breathing involves inhaling through the nose and lifting the diaphragm at the top of the abdomen. Some people tend to over-breathe (hyperventilate) when they are feeling anxious. Their breathing tends to be rapid and shallow, and is via the mouth. This type of breathing leads to more air finding its way down the gullet and into the stomach, where it causes wind, bloating, rumbling and pain.

14 Identify whether you swallow air when anxious

Next time you're feeling anxious, check how you are breathing. If you are breathing through your nose and expanding your stomach first and then your chest, you are a 'normal' breather. If you notice you are breathing quickly through your mouth and expanding your chest first and then your stomach only slightly, or not at all, you are an 'over-breather'. If you recognise yourself as an 'over-breather', practising normal abdominal breathing may help. This type of breathing is also an instant de-stresser when you can feel your tension levels rising.

15 Practise abdominal breathing

1. Make sure you are sitting comfortably with your shoulders lowered and relaxed.

2. Inhale slowly through both nostrils to a count of five, expanding your tummy.

3. Hold for 5 seconds and then exhale to a count of five, drawing your tummy in.

16 Determine whether your emotions are affecting your gut

To determine whether stress is affecting your digestive system, record your IBS symptoms for at least one month. Alongside the symptoms, rate, from zero to ten, how stressed/anxious/depressed you are feeling, with zero being 'not stressed/anxious/depressed at all' and ten being 'extremely stressed/anxious/depressed'. If you notice a link between your emotions and your IBS symptoms, you could benefit from taking steps to manage your stress levels and mood. There are basically three things you can do about stress: avoid it, reduce it and relieve it.

17 Keep a stress diary

Over a couple of weeks, note down the details of situations, times, places and people that make you feel stressed. Once you've identified these, you need to think about each one and ask yourself: 'Can I avoid it?' For example, if driving to work during the rush hour makes you feel extremely stressed, perhaps you can avoid doing it by starting or finishing work a little earlier or later? If you cannot avoid it, you can usually reduce the level of stress you experience by changing your attitude or by taking practical steps to help you cope better. You can also relieve the effects of stress by practising relaxation techniques and doing things that help you unwind.

18 Value what you already have

As well as recognising the external factors that make you feel stressed, consider whether some aspects of your personality are also to blame. Are you a perfectionist who is never satisfied with your achievements and lifestyle? Constantly feeling that who you are and what you have aren't good enough can lead to unrealistic expectations, discontent and unnecessary pressure. Instead, learn to value your accomplishments and what you already have. In his best-selling book *Don't Sweat the Small Stuff*, Dr Richard Carlson urges us to remind ourselves that 'life is okay the way it is, right now'. Adopting this attitude immediately reduces stress and induces calm.

⑲ Remember that you'll never reach the end of your to-do list

Workaholism is another factor that tends to be linked with perfectionism – a 'perfect' home and lifestyle have to be paid for. While working hard for what you want in life is commendable, some people work such long hours that they don't have time to enjoy what they have. If you're constantly driven to get everything done, and think you'll feel calm and relaxed once everything on your to-do list is completed, think again! What tends to happen is that as you complete tasks, you add new ones to your list, so you never get to the end of it. It's a fact of life that there will always be tasks to be completed. Dr Carlson suggests you remind yourself that, when you die, you will leave behind unfinished business!

⑳ Develop a positive attitude

Changing your attitude towards difficult situations can reduce the amount of stress they cause. When something bad happens, instead of thinking about how awful the situation is, try to find something positive about it if you can. Try to find answers to your problems, or view them as an opportunity for personal growth. For example, being made redundant initially might seem like a negative event but, if you view it as an opportunity to retrain and start a new career doing something you really enjoy, it can become a catalyst for positive change.

21 Live in the moment

Living in the moment, or practising mindfulness, has been shown to reduce stress levels. It involves giving all of your attention to the here and now, rather than worrying about the past or future, and has its roots in Buddhism. It's based on the philosophy that you can't alter the past, or foretell the future, but you can influence what's happening in your life right now. By living fully in the present, you can perform to the best of your ability, whereas worrying about the past and future can hamper how you function now, and increase your stress levels unnecessarily.

In his book *Stop Thinking, Start Living*, Dr Carlson suggests that anxiety and depression are the result of dwelling on the past or thinking about the future and that the way to healthy mental functioning is to focus your attention on the present.

Living in this way means your experience of life is richer, because instead of doing things on autopilot, all of your senses will be fully engaged in what you are doing. Imagine going for a walk in the park while being so preoccupied with worries about the future, or regrets about the past, that you don't even notice your surroundings. Then think how much more pleasurable and relaxing the experience would be if you took the time to absorb the sights, sounds and smells around you. When you focus on the here and now, you will find yourself appreciating the simple things in your life more.

Mindfulness is also about being happy with your life as it is now, rather than thinking you can only be happy when you've achieved certain things – such as a better job, or a bigger house or bank balance. Adopting this attitude towards life will immediately lower your stress levels. If you find it hard to focus on the present, try keeping a daily diary.

Dr Carlson also claims that problems become easier to solve when you focus on what actions you can take now to resolve them. Even taking the tiniest step towards a solution today can make you feel better and more in control of your situation, which in turn reduces stress levels. You can also develop your ability to focus on the present by practising simple meditation, which is discussed a little further on in this chapter.

Prioritise

When you have a long to-do list, number tasks in terms of urgency and importance, and carry them out in that order.

22 Learn to delegate

Perfectionism can also lead to a need to control – you convince yourself that no one else can meet your high standards and so you do everything yourself. This inevitably leads to physical and mental overload. The solution is to accept that you can't know and do everything, so you need to learn to listen to other people's ideas and opinions and to delegate. Ask your partner and children to help with domestic tasks and accept any offers of help at work.

23 Simplify your life

If a bulging wardrobe, heaving shelves and overflowing cupboards are getting you down, make your life simpler and less stressful by getting rid of unnecessary clutter around your home. If you haven't worn, read or used an item for two years or more, give it to a charity shop, or bin it. If you can't bear to get rid of it, store it in the loft, then make it a rule that if you haven't thought about using the item within six months it is time to part with it. If you have a lot of possessions to sort out, ask your partner, a family member or a friend to help you. You'll be amazed at how much lighter and happier you will feel after a good clear out.

If you feel that your life is spiralling out of control with too many demands from work, your home, your partner, and your family and friends, maybe it's time to simplify your life. If you regularly feel under pressure and stressed because of a lack of time, try reviewing how you use it. Keep a diary for a few days to see how you spend your time and then decide which activities you can cut out or reduce to make more time for the things that are most important to you. Try saying 'no' to the non-essential tasks you don't have time for, or just don't want to do. It's a little word, but it can dramatically reduce your stress levels. If you find it hard to say 'no', then perhaps you need to develop your assertiveness skills.

24 Be assertive

If you feel you often hide your true feelings, instead of expressing them, and give in to others to gain their approval, or so that you don't hurt or upset them, you might benefit from brushing up on your assertiveness skills.

Do you regularly allow others to manipulate you into doing things you don't want to do? Being assertive enables you to say what you want, feel and need, calmly and confidently, without being aggressive or hurting others. Try the following techniques to develop your self-assertiveness, so that you remain in control of your life and do things because you want to, rather than to please other people.

Demonstrate ownership of your thoughts, feelings and behaviour by using 'I' rather than 'we', 'you' or 'it'. So rather than saying 'You make me angry', try something like 'I feel angry when you…'. This is also less antagonising to the other person.

When you have a choice whether to do something or not, say 'won't' rather than 'can't' to indicate that you've made an active decision, rather than suggesting that something or someone has stopped you. Say 'choose to' instead of 'have to' and 'could' rather than 'should', to show that you have a choice. For example: 'I won't be going out tonight' rather than 'I can't go out tonight' or ' I could go out tonight, but I have chosen to stay in'.

When you feel that your needs aren't being considered, state what you want calmly and clearly, repeating it until the other person shows they've heard and understood what you've said.

When making a request, identify exactly what it is you want and what you're prepared to settle for. Choose positive, assertive words, as outlined above. For example: 'I would like you to help me tidy the kitchen' or 'I'd really appreciate it if you could empty the kitchen bin'.

When refusing a request, speak calmly but firmly, giving the reason or reasons why, without apologising. Repeat if you need to. For example: 'I won't be able to babysit for you tonight because I'm feeling really tired after being at work all day.'

When you disagree with someone, say so using the word 'I'. Explain why you disagree, while acknowledging the other person's right to hold a different viewpoint. For example: 'I don't agree that the service in that restaurant is poor – our meal was only late last time we visited because it was extremely busy, but I can understand why you think that.'

25 Find social support

IBS can be an isolating and embarrassing condition and many sufferers feel that no one understands what they are experiencing. Making contact with fellow sufferers may help you overcome these feelings – the following organisations offer the opportunity to do just that. Further information and contact details are listed in the Directory at the end of the book:

The Bladder and Bowel Foundation is a charity providing information and support for those with bladder or bowel problems and offers an online forum and chat room.

The IBS Network offers its members a network of self-help groups, as well as a helpline, befriender penfriend schemes and online forums.

The Irritable Bowel Syndrome Self Help and Support Group is a US website that was launched in 1995 and claims to be the largest community for IBS sufferers, with over 62,350 active members and 800,000 postings. The site offers forums, blogs, a chat room and a pen pals list.

IBS Tales is a website set up by an IBS sufferer called Sophie, who has had the condition for over 20 years. The site offers sufferers the opportunity to read about others' experiences and write about their own if they wish. Sophie also writes an online blog about IBS.

26 Sleep well

Sleep is a factor in IBS: too little sleep or sleep of poor quality have both been shown to have a direct effect on the severity of IBS symptoms the following morning, probably because they increase stress levels.

To sleep more soundly, try the following strategies:

- Get outdoors during the day. Exposure to daylight stops the production of melatonin, the brain chemical that promotes sleep, making it easier for your body to release it at night so that you fall asleep more easily and sleep more soundly.

- Choose foods rich in tryptophan, an amino acid your body uses to produce serotonin (a brain chemical that's converted into the 'sleep hormone' melatonin). Tryptophan-rich foods include bananas, dates, dairy foods, chicken, turkey, rice, oats, wholegrain breads and cereals. An added bonus is that, if you suffer from constipation, these foods could help, as increasing your serotonin levels will increase your gut motility.

- Make sure you're neither too hungry nor too full when you go to bed, as both can cause wakefulness.

- Don't drink coffee or cola after 2 p.m. because the stimulant effects of the caffeine they contain can last for hours. While tea contains about half as much caffeine – around 50 mg per cup – it's best not to drink it near bedtime if you have difficulty sleeping. Redbush or herbal teas, which are caffeine-free, make good alternatives.

- Exercise can help you sleep more soundly, because it encourages your body temperature and metabolism to increase and then fall a few hours later, which promotes sleep. Try not to exercise later than early evening: exercising too late at night can have the opposite effect, because the body temperature may still be raised at bedtime. Not taking enough exercise can cause sleep problems and restlessness.

- Wind down before bedtime. Develop a regular routine in the evening that allows you to 'put the day to bed'. This could involve watching TV – if you find that relaxing – though it's probably best to avoid watching anything that could prey on your mind later on when you are trying to go to sleep. Other relaxing activities you could do include reading – though it's best to avoid over-stimulating books – listening to music and having a long soak in a warm bath.

- Avoid drinking alcohol at bedtime: although it may relax you at first and help you fall asleep more quickly, it has a stimulant effect, causing you to wake more during the night. It's also a diuretic, making nocturnal trips to the toilet more likely. But, if abstinence doesn't help you sleep better, it may be worth indulging in a glass of Cabernet Sauvignon, Merlot or Chianti at bedtime – there's some evidence that these wines improve your sleep patterns because the grape skins they contain are rich in plant melatonin.

- Ensure your bedroom is cool and dark. Your brain tries to reduce your body temperature at night to slow down your metabolism. So to encourage sleep, aim for a temperature of around 16°C. Darkness stimulates the pineal gland in the brain to produce melatonin.

- To help your brain associate the bedroom with sleep and sex only, avoid having a TV, computer or other digital device in your bedroom. Watching action-packed TV programmes or using a digital device last thing at night can overstimulate your brain, making it harder for you to switch off and fall asleep. Also, both TV and computer screens emit bright light that may decrease the production of melatonin – however, watching TV in the dark can help reduce the effects.

- Only go to bed when you feel really sleepy. If you can't drop off within what seems like about 20 minutes, get up and do something you find relaxing, but not too stimulating, such as reading or listening to calming music. Only return to your bed when you feel sleepy again – this helps to reinforce your brain's connection between your bed and sleep.

- Soak in a warm bath at bedtime. Your temperature increases slightly with the warmth and then falls – helping you to drop off. Add a few drops of essential oils, such as lavender or camomile, for their soothing properties.

- If mulling over problems or a busy schedule the next day stops you from falling asleep, try writing down your concerns or a plan for the day ahead before you go to bed.

Make time to unwind

Spend some of the time you've saved by simplifying your life doing something purely for pleasure, whether it's luxuriating in a hot, scented bath with a glass of wine and a good book, listening to your favourite music, or going to the cinema to see a film. Doing something you really enjoy will help take your mind off domestic and work pressures.

27 Have a hug

Research suggests that having regular hugs reduces stress hormones in the bloodstream and lowers blood pressure.

28 Laugh more

Laughter is a great stress reliever. A good belly laugh seems to reduce the stress hormones cortisol and adrenaline, and increase mood-boosting serotonin levels. People who see the funny side of life appear to have a reduced risk of the health problems associated with stress. So make time to watch your favourite comedies and comedians, and be around people who make you laugh. Or, visit www.laughlab.co.uk or www.ahajokes.com whenever you feel like a good giggle!

29 Get physical!

Regular exercise is a great antidote to stress because it enables the body to utilise the stress hormones whose original purpose was to provide the extra energy needed to run away from our aggressors, or to stay put and fight. It also triggers the release of endorphins, which act as natural painkillers and antidepressants.

In 2008, researchers from the University of Birmingham confirmed that findings from other studies indicating that regular exercise reduced bloating and constipation in IBS sufferers were correct. It seems that regular exercise stimulates gut contractions and that a couch potato lifestyle can make the gut lazy.

One group of IBS sufferers was encouraged to do 30 minutes of moderate-intensity exercise (e.g. brisk walking or yoga) five times a week and had two personalised exercise consultations to motivate and inform them. A second group was offered standard

IBS treatment and lifestyle advice. After three months, the participants who were encouraged to exercise were found to have been more active than the other group, and they reported greater improvements in their symptoms, especially constipation.

Another study at the University of British Columbia in Vancouver found yoga to be especially beneficial for IBS sufferers (see chapter 8). Swimming is another moderate-intensity exercise that may be worth trying. For information about swimming lessons, visit www.swimtime.org. To improve your swimming technique from your desk, visit www.swimfit.com, a website that offers animated swimming stroke guides. T'ai chi, described as a 'moving meditation', may also help. For classes near you, visit www.taichifinder.co.uk.

However, you don't need to join a class to become more active; incorporating exercise into your daily routine is easy and effective. Putting more effort into the housework and gardening, walking the dog, getting up from your desk and walking around regularly, and walking while talking on your mobile are all ways of being more active.

30 Try ecotherapy

Researchers at the University of Essex say that ecotherapy (engaging with nature) offers both mental and physical health benefits. Whether through an active pursuit, such as walking or gardening, or a passive one, like admiring the view, being close to nature has been shown to reduce stress and ease muscular tension. Experts believe that the higher levels of negative ions near areas with running water, trees and mountains may play a part. Others claim that the success of ecotherapy is down to biophilia and had the theory that we have an innate affinity with nature and that our 'disconnection' from it is the cause of stress and mental health problems. Studies in the Netherlands and Japan suggest that people living in or near green areas enjoy a longer and healthier life than those living in urban environments.

31 Relax your muscles

The progressive muscle relaxation technique helps to release tension from the muscles. According to Richard Hilliard, director of the Relaxation for Living Institute (RFLI), it's impossible to have an anxious mind when your muscles are relaxed. The institute's website offers advice on relaxation and stress management.

Try following these steps whenever you feel tense and anxious:

- Take a deep breath and then create tension in your face by clenching your teeth and screwing up your eyes tightly, then relax and breathe out.

- Take a deep breath, then lift the muscles in your shoulders, tense them for a few seconds and then relax, dropping your shoulders and releasing the tension as you breathe out.

- Take a deep breath, then clench your fists and tense the muscles in your arms, hold for a few seconds, then release and breathe out.

- Next, tense the muscles in your buttocks and both of your legs, including the thighs and calves, hold, and then release as you breathe out.

- Finally, clench your toes and tense your feet, hold, and then release and breathe out.

Alternatively, you can buy a guide to deep relaxation as an MP3 download on the RFLI website (see Directory).

32 Meditate

Research suggests that meditation lowers stress hormones. Since IBS is linked to stress, it's not surprising that a study suggested that meditation helps to reduce symptoms such as pain and bloating. Participants in the study learned how to meditate at six weekly classes. After a year of practising meditation, eight out of ten people reported that their symptoms had improved.

There are various meditation techniques, but here is a simple one that can be practised whenever you have a few moments to yourself – even while you are on the bus or train!

- Close your eyes and focus on your breathing.

- As you inhale slowly and deeply through your nose, expand your stomach, and hold for a few seconds, before drawing in your stomach, while exhaling slowly.

- Whenever your attention is distracted by a passing thought, return to simply observing your breathing.

- If you prefer, you can listen to a step-by-step mindfulness meditation at www.stressmanagement.co.uk.

> ### Try complementary therapies
> Various complementary therapies, including acupressure, aromatherapy, massage, reflexology and yoga, are thought to help relieve psychological stress and muscle tension. For ideas on how you can practise these therapies at home, see chapter 8.

33 Seek help

Finally, don't be afraid to ask for professional help if you feel you can't deal with life's stresses on your own. Your first port of call should be your doctor, as he or she will be able to offer advice and possibly refer you to a trained counsellor.

The Stress Management Society offers further guidance on dealing with stress, including 'desk yoga' and 'desk massage' techniques you can practise at work, and a creative visualisation you can do when you have a few minutes to yourself. See the Directory at the end of the book for contact details.

Chapter 5

Hormones and IBS

One explanation for more women than men suffering from IBS is that the female hormones oestrogen and progesterone are somehow implicated in their symptoms. Receptors (proteins on the surface of cells), designed to bind with and react to these hormones, have been found in the gut lining, suggesting that they may have a role in regulating the way the gut functions. Many women experience gastrointestinal changes at times in their cycle when levels of these hormones fluctuate the most.

Up to 45 per cent of women with IBS find that their symptoms get worse just before and during the early part of their monthly period. Around a third of women who don't suffer from IBS also experience changes in their bowel habits at this time in their cycle. Research suggests that there could be a number of reasons for this. For example, both oestrogen and progesterone seem to have a relaxant effect on the muscles in the gut, which is why food transit time is slower in women than in men. Oestrogen and progesterone levels are high during the second half of the menstrual cycle (after ovulation), so the speed at which food is pushed through the digestive system is much slower, making constipation more likely. Just before a period and for the first couple of days, progesterone and oestrogen levels are at their lowest, so gut contractions speed up, resulting in diarrhoea and cramping pains. As the ovaries begin to release more and more oestrogen to thicken the uterus prior to ovulation, these symptoms subside again.

It's also likely that the prostaglandins (hormone-like chemicals), released by the uterus to stimulate the contractions that expel the womb lining, also speed up gut contractions, leading to cramping pains and diarrhoea. Added to this, studies suggest that women with IBS may be more sensitive to intestinal pain during their periods.

Another theory is that increased progesterone levels during the latter half of the menstrual cycle may increase bacterial activity in the gut, leading to wind, bloating and diarrhoea.

PMS (Premenstrual Syndrome) in the week or so before a period can cause psychological symptoms, such as tension and mood swings, which can also affect how the gut functions. Studies suggest that women with IBS tend to suffer from the most severe premenstrual symptoms, such as bloating and difficulty in concentrating.

34 Keep a diary

The easiest way to determine whether your IBS symptoms are made worse by shifts in your hormone levels is to keep a diary over at least three cycles. An easy way to do this is to simply mark the dates of your period with a tick. Highlight the days you suffer from IBS symptoms with a cross, and note down the symptoms and their severity. It may help if you rate your symptoms out of ten – with one being the least severe and ten being the most. That way you can see at a glance when your symptoms are at their worst, and whether they coincide with the days just before and early on in your period. If you tend to suffer from IBS-C, you may notice that your constipation gets progressively worse after ovulation, but then improves at the onset of your period. On the other hand, if you suffer from IBS-D, you may notice exactly the opposite effect, with your symptoms improving after ovulation, and worsening just before and for the first couple of days of menstruation.

If you have noticed a link between your menstrual cycle and your symptoms, there are steps you can take to lessen the effects.

35 Be prepared (IBS-A and IBS-D)

If you have IBS-A or IBS-D, you can take these extra precautions a few days before your period is due, until a couple of days after it starts:

- Be especially careful about what you eat, and make sure you avoid any food triggers.

- Cut back on foods containing insoluble fibre and artificial sweeteners.

- Try eating foods high in calcium, such as dairy foods.

If dairy foods trigger your symptoms, green leafy vegetables, nuts, tinned sardines with the bones, dried apricots, almonds and Brazil nuts are good alternatives. This can help in two ways: calcium levels appear to drop at menstruation and eating calcium-rich foods appears to help reduce PMS. Calcium also seems to slow down gut contractions, reducing diarrhoea.

If you think PMS may be exacerbating your symptoms, try taking a supplement that can help, such as agnus castus or evening primrose oil. In one controlled trial of women whose IBS was related to their menstrual cycle, over half reported an improvement after taking evening primrose oil. You can also buy commercial formulae specifically for PMS, such as FemmeVit, (see Useful Products at the end of the book).

To reduce the risk of PMS, be especially aware of your stress levels in the week or so before your period is due. Try to lighten your workload as much as possible and follow the stress management tips outlined in chapter 4.

36 Be prepared (IBS-C)

If you suffer from IBS-C, there are steps you can take during the second half of your cycle to counteract the constipating effects of progesterone and oestrogen:

- Make sure you drink plenty of water
- Eat more fibre-rich foods, or take a fibre supplement
- Fit more exercise into your daily life.

Chapter 6

Medications for IBS

While the aim of this book is to help you control your IBS by identifying and reducing your triggers, and using natural supplements and stress management techniques, it's still a good idea to have effective treatments to help you deal with your symptoms if and when they strike. In addition, if, despite making changes to your diet and lifestyle, your symptoms persist, medications may be advised.

There are a variety of over-the-counter and prescription-only treatments that you can try, depending on your symptoms. The three main ones are antispasmodics to alleviate cramping pains, antimotility drugs to treat diarrhoea, and laxatives to relieve constipation. Antidepressants, such as tricyclics, are sometimes prescribed to relieve persistent abdominal pain, and selective serotonin reuptake inhibitors (SSRIs) may be prescribed where constipation is also a symptom. As well as having beneficial effects, most medicines can cause unwanted side effects – though not everyone experiences them.

37 Try an antispasmodic to relieve abdominal pain and cramps

Antispasmodics relax the smooth muscle in the gut lining to prevent and relieve painful cramps. Smooth muscle is a type of muscle that you can't control voluntarily.

There are two types of antispasmodics:

- Direct-acting smooth muscle relaxants, such as peppermint oil, alverine and mebeverine
- Antimuscarinics (also known as anticholinergics), such as hyoscine butylbromide and dicycloverine.

Peppermint oil, alverine and mebeverine mainly act on smooth intestinal muscle, so they have relatively few adverse effects. Antimuscarinics, such as hyoscine butylbromide, are less selective, which means they are more likely to affect other parts of the body and cause adverse effects.

Colpermin

Colpermin is an over-the-counter and prescription antispasmodic drug containing peppermint oil. It's available in capsule form, with an enteric coating that enables it to remain whole until it reaches the intestines, where it begins to dissolve. As the peppermint oil is released, it relaxes any spasms in the intestinal walls, allowing trapped wind to escape. Colpermin is usually well tolerated, though if you suffer from heartburn it may make it worse. It can occasionally irritate the area around the bottom, and, in extremely rare cases, the menthol in the drug could cause an allergic reaction. Mintec is another antispasmodic that contains peppermint oil.

Spasmonal

Spasmonal capsules contain the active ingredient alverine citrate, which is a type of smooth muscle relaxant. Alverine is available as a capsule both on prescription and over the counter. If you are pregnant or breastfeeding, consult your GP or pharmacist before taking them. Side effects are usually mild and can include nausea, headaches, dizziness and, on rare occasions, signs of allergy, such as a rash, itching or shortness of breath.

Colofac IBS

Colofac IBS is a prescription-only antispasmodic that contains mebeverine hydrochloride, which works by relaxing the smooth muscle in the gut. The tablets are usually taken three times daily, about 20 minutes before a meal. This medicine should be used with caution during pregnancy and breastfeeding, and by those with hereditary blood disorders, known as porphyria. On rare occasions, it causes allergic reactions, such as rashes, hives (itchy swollen areas of skin) or severe swelling of the lips, tongue or face. Mebeverine is also available as a generic medicine (i.e. without a brand name).

Buscopan

Buscopan is an over-the-counter antispasmodic. Its active ingredient is hyoscine butylbromide, which is derived from the leaves of the Australian tree known as the corkwood tree or

Duboisia. A relative of this tree, the datura, was used by ancient Hindu physicians as an antispasmodic. It works by interrupting the brain signals that 'tell' the muscles to cramp, so that the muscles can relax and return to normal. This drug is usually well tolerated, however, up to one in ten users experience a dry mouth. Less common side effects include skin reactions, increased heart rate, difficulty in breathing, reduced sweat production, inability to pass urine, and allergic reactions, which can be severe.

38 Try an antimotility drug for IBS-D

Antimotility drugs are useful for treating diarrhoea. They work by slowing down gut contractions (motility), thus reducing the speed at which food passes through the digestive system. Because the food remains in the intestines for longer, more water is absorbed back into the body, resulting in firmer stools that need to be passed less often.

Commonly used antimotility drugs include:

Loperamide
Loperamide is the most commonly used antimotility drug for treating diarrhoea in IBS. Although it's an opiate, it is unlikely to cause dependence, but should still be used with caution. Some people take loperamide only when they need it, while others take it regularly as a precautionary measure, especially prior to situations that might bring on an attack, or where finding a loo may

be a problem. Possible side effects include tummy cramps and bloating, a skin rash, itching, dizziness, drowsiness and nausea. Speak to your GP or pharmacist if you experience these or other side effects. Over-the-counter medications containing loperamide include Imodium, Diocalm, Entrocalm, Norimode and Normaloe.

Lomotil

Lomotil is a prescription-only antimotility drug. It contains the opiate diphenoxylate, and atropine sulphate. Diphenoxylate blocks the nerve signals to the intestinal muscles, relaxing the muscles and reducing contractions. This slows the passage of food through the gut, so that more water is absorbed from food remains and bowel movements are firmer and fewer. Diphenoxylate also relieves painful muscle contractions and prevents spasms. Atropine sulphate blocks nerve signals to the bowel muscles so that they relax, preventing spasms. Lomotil should be used with caution during pregnancy and breastfeeding, and by those with heart problems, decreased kidney function, liver disease, ulcerative colitis or Down's syndrome. It should be avoided by people with glaucoma, and those taking a type of antidepressant called monoamine oxidase inhibitors (MAOIs). Lomotil should be taken with plenty of water. Possible side effects include dry mouth and thirst, flushing, irregular heartbeat and constipation. Long-term use of this drug is not recommended because it can cause dependency.

39 Try laxatives for IBS-C

Your doctor may advise laxatives if you have constipation-predominant IBS and find it difficult to include sufficient fibre in your diet, or if you experience excessive wind and bloating when you eat fibre-rich foods. There are three types of laxative, and each relieves constipation in a different way. Bulk-forming laxatives soften and 'bulk up' faeces, encouraging your bowels to move and push the faeces out. Osmotic laxatives increase the amount of water that stays in your faeces as they pass through your intestines, making them softer and easier to pass. Stimulant laxatives work by speeding up intestinal contractions and should only be used occasionally because the bowel can become dependent on them.

Bulk-forming laxatives include:

Sterculia

Sterculia is a vegetable gum from the karaya tree that is used as a bulk-forming laxative to treat constipation. It can absorb up to 60 times its own volume in water. Although it's less likely to be fermented by bacteria in the gut than wheat bran, it may still cause wind and bloating in some people. It's available over the counter and on prescription in granule form as Normacol. You can take the granules with water or stir them into foods like yogurt.

Ispaghula husk

Ispaghula husk is available as an over-the-counter and prescription medication in powder and granule form. This medication forms a gel when it mixes with fluid, which softens and bulks up the stools and stimulates gut contractions. It must be taken with sufficient water. Some people experience wind and bloating when taking ispaghula. This may decrease over time – if not, speak to your GP or pharmacist. Over-the-counter products containing ispaghula include Fybogel (orange-flavoured granules you add to water) and Isogel (mint granules you swallow with water). Your GP may prescribe a generic (non-branded) ispaghula. See also under Supplements in chapter 3.

Methylcellulose

Methylcellulose is a plant fibre that is helpful both for sufferers of diarrhoea and constipation. It isn't absorbed into the bloodstream, but stays in the intestines, where it absorbs water and swells up to form a gel. With diarrhoea, it adds bulk to the stool and, with constipation, it makes stools softer and easier to pass. It shouldn't be taken by people with bowel infections or blockages. It appears to be safe for use during pregnancy and breastfeeding, and no side effects have been reported. An over-the-counter brand name is Celevac.

Commonly used osmotic laxatives include:

Milk of Magnesia

Milk of Magnesia contains magnesium hydroxide, which helps to prevent the bowels from reabsorbing water from the stools, so that they are softer and passed more readily. You must drink plenty of fluids with this treatment and you should stop taking this medicine if you experience diarrhoea. You shouldn't take it for more than three consecutive days. Milk of Magnesia can cross the placenta and pass into breast milk, so its use should be avoided during pregnancy and breastfeeding.

Movicol

Movicol is a prescription-only osmotic laxative that contains macrogol, sodium bicarbonate, sodium chloride and potassium chloride. Macrogol causes the water that it is taken with to be retained in the intestine rather than absorbed, making the stools softer and easier to pass. The sodium bicarbonate, sodium chloride and potassium chloride (electrolytes) are included in this medicine to help ensure that the laxative works without causing the body to gain or lose significant amounts of sodium, potassium or water. However, prolonged use for the treatment of constipation in IBS is not recommended. Those with heart disease should use it with caution. Anyone who feels weak, fatigued, breathless or thirsty, has a headache, or gets swollen ankles, should stop taking this medication and consult their GP, as these symptoms may indicate that the levels of minerals that control your fluid balance (electrolytes) are disturbed.

Stimulant laxatives include:

Bisacodyl

Bisacodyl is available on prescription and as the over-the-counter medication Dulcolax. Bisacodyl works by stimulating the nerve endings in the walls of the large intestine and rectum, making them contract more often and more forcefully, relieving constipation. Bisacodyl tablets have an enteric coating to prevent them from dissolving in the acidic environment of the stomach, so that they dissolve in the large intestine instead. They start to work within 6 to 12 hours and should therefore be taken at night to provide relief from constipation the next morning. This medication shouldn't be taken continuously for more than five days, as it may cause diarrhoea and an imbalance of fluids and electrolytes. People with a blockage in the gut shouldn't take it. Bisacodyl appears to be safe for use during pregnancy and breastfeeding, but consult your pharmacist or GP before taking this medication, as they may suggest gentler alternatives.

Senna

Senna has traditionally been used to treat constipation in India and North Africa. It works by stimulating the nerve endings in the walls of the large intestine and rectum, increasing the frequency and strength of their contractions, and relieving constipation. Senna contains sennosides, which are activated by gut bacteria and, because they increase gut contractions, they can cause stomach cramps. If you don't have a bowel movement within three days of taking senna, see your GP. Don't take it for longer than seven days, as prolonged use may cause the gut to become over-reliant on its use. People with a blockage of the gut should not take this medicine. Senna is believed to be safe for use during pregnancy and breastfeeding, but consult your pharmacist or GP first, as there may be gentler alternatives. Senokot is a popular brand of over-the-counter products containing senna. The range includes both tablets and syrup (see Useful Products).

40 Ask your GP about taking antidepressants

If your symptoms persist despite lifestyle and dietary changes, your GP may suggest a low dose (10 mg) of an antidepressant to be taken at night to ease abdominal pain and other symptoms. Antidepressants are thought to work by blocking pain signals to the brain, and seem to be especially helpful during times of stress – possibly because they ease any underlying anxiety and depression, which might play a part in some people's IBS symptoms. There are two main types of antidepressant your GP might prescribe, depending on your symptoms: tricyclics and selective serotonin reuptake inhibitors (SSRIs). Like any medication, antidepressants can cause side effects, so it is advisable to view them as a short-term solution only.

If you would prefer not to take medications, you might consider trying the herbal remedy St John's wort instead. Research suggests it is as effective as mild antidepressants for the treatment of mild to moderate depression.

If you're taking any kind of medication, speak to your pharmacist or GP before using St John's wort, as it can interact with several commonly prescribed drugs, including oral contraceptives, anti-epileptic drugs, warfarin and the antibiotic tetracycline. It can also increase sensitivity to sunlight.

Tricyclics

If you have diarrhoea-predominant symptoms, your GP may offer tricyclic antidepressants, such as amitriptyline or trimipramine, because a common side effect of these drugs is constipation, which means they can help treat diarrhoea, as well as abdominal pain. Other common side effects include drowsiness, dry mouth, blurred vision, increased appetite and weight gain. Relatively uncommon side effects include nausea, headache and palpitations. Note: tricyclics may pose a risk to a developing baby in the womb, so if you discover you are pregnant you should discuss the risks and benefits with your GP.

Selective serotonin reuptake inhibitors (SSRIs)

If you suffer from chronic constipation-predominant IBS, your GP may advise a type of antidepressant called selective serotonin reuptake inhibitors (SSRIs), of which the most well known are probably Prozac and Seroxat. SSRIs increase serotonin levels by preventing the reuptake of serotonin by nerve cells in the brain. One of the roles of serotonin is to regulate gut contractions – higher levels increase the number of contractions – which is beneficial if you suffer from constipation. However, if you suffer from diarrhoea-predominant IBS, SSRIs should not be prescribed, as they could worsen your symptoms. As well as diarrhoea, other possible side effects include nausea, loss of appetite, dry mouth and headache. These should settle down within one to two weeks – if they don't you should see your GP.

It is worth ensuring your diet contains enough serotonin-producing foods, before trying medications with potential side effects (see Sleep well on pp.92–95).

Note

This is not a comprehensive list of medications for IBS. Always read the guidance leaflet when taking any medication. For details of other suitable medications, speak to your GP or pharmacist.

Chapter 7

Living with IBS

Suffering from IBS can make everyday-living difficult – always having to be able to find a loo and being careful about what you eat can make eating out and travelling especially trying. This chapter offers practical tips to help you plan ahead, so that you can stop worrying about your symptoms and relax and enjoy yourself.

41 Enjoy eating out

Eating out can be a nerve-wracking experience if you suffer from IBS. Many sufferers find that eating triggers their symptoms. You may be concerned about having to avoid your food triggers and finding the loo. Plan beforehand with the following tips to help make the experience less fraught.

Find the loo
Check where the loo is as soon as possible after you arrive. This will help you feel less concerned if you need to dash to it later on.

Access the menu beforehand

Try to access the menu beforehand, so that you can plan your selection in advance. Many restaurants now have their own website displaying the menu details. Opt for foods you know are safe. If you're unsure about any of the ingredients, you can ring up beforehand to ask what they are. If that's not possible, ask the waiter prior to ordering. Some restaurants might be happy to modify a recipe if you ask. For example, you could ask them to use less chilli in a curry, etc.

Pre-medicate

If you know that eating out will almost certainly trigger an attack of IBS symptoms, take a preventative dose of medication, such as an antidiarrhoeal or antispasmodic, before you go out.

Try not to overeat

Eating too much might trigger your symptoms. Avoid large portions, or stick to just one or two courses. Some restaurants may be happy to serve smaller portions if you ask.

Relax!

Worrying about your symptoms will make you more at risk of suffering an attack, so remember to relax and enjoy the company, food and surroundings! Try doing some deep breathing exercises before you set off in order to keep anxiety at bay (see chapter 4, p.84).

42 Travel without worry

Travelling can be especially worrying if you have IBS. Sitting for long periods, motion sickness, anxiety about finding a loo, eating strange foods and having your sleep patterns disrupted can potentially worsen IBS symptoms. Needing to visit the loo several times while driving, or travelling by bus or by train, is often inconvenient, embarrassing and possibly unpleasant, depending on the state of the conveniences provided. Even a short-haul flight can be an ordeal if you have a bout of diarrhoea. However, there are a few things you can do to reduce the chances of an attack and to help you cope if you do develop IBS symptoms during your journey.

Watch what you eat before and during the journey

Try not to eat too much just before your journey. Choose plain food that is less likely to irritate your gut. If you're flying and are concerned that the in-flight meal might trigger your symptoms, carry a suitable snack in your hand luggage.

Drink plenty of water

Drinking plenty of water during the trip is important for those with IBS-C, in order to keep the gut functioning properly, and for those with IBS-D, in order to replace lost fluids.

Avoid 'traveller's tummy'

Make sure you don't exacerbate your symptoms by picking up a tummy infection. Wash your hands frequently – carrying a handsanitising gel with you is a good precaution in case there are no, or inadequate, handwashing facilities during your trip. Drink only bottled water while abroad. Avoid eating undercooked fish or meat, and check that an establishment looks clean before eating there.

Locate the nearest loo

When travelling by bus, train or plane, make sure you locate the nearest loo as soon as you get on board.

If you're travelling in the UK, the Great British Public Toilet website: www.greatbritishpublictoiletmap.rca.ac.uk offers an online 'loo locator' to help you find out beforehand where public toilets are located at your destination – always useful to know in case you need to find one in a hurry. It might also be a good idea to buy a RADAR key, which enables you to access around 9,000 locked disabled toilets across the UK. These are available from Disability Rights UK. See Useful Products for further details.

Carry an emergency kit

Carry an emergency kit with you, so that you are prepared if you have an attack. It could consist of an easy-to-take antidiarrhoeal (such as Imodium Instant Melts, which don't require water), wet wipes, tissues, a spare set of pants, panty liners or incontinence pads and a fragranced body spray.

Chapter 8

DIY
Complementary
Therapies

The main difference between complementary therapies (also known as alternative, natural or holistic therapies) and conventional Western medicine is that the former approach focuses on treating the individual as a whole, whereas the latter is symptom-led. Complementary practitioners view illness as a sign that physical and mental well-being have been disrupted, and they attempt to restore good health by stimulating the body's own self-healing and self-regulating abilities. They claim that total well-being can be achieved when the mind and body are in a state of balance called homeostasis. Homeostasis is achieved by following the type of lifestyle advocated in this book, i.e. a healthy diet with plenty of fresh air, exercise, sleep and relaxation, combined with stress management and a positive mental attitude.

Whether complementary therapies work or not remains under debate. Some argue that any benefits are a result of the placebo effect. This is where a treatment brings about improvements simply because the person using it expects it to, rather than because it has any real effect. However, it could be argued that, unlike drug treatments, which are comparatively recent, complementary therapies like aromatherapy, massage and reflexology have stood the test of time, having been used to treat ailments and promote well-being for thousands of years. The use of complementary therapies alongside conventional medicine received an unexpected boost when the National Institute for Health and Care Excellence (NICE) recommended acupuncture and chiropractic treatments, along with exercise therapy, for the treatment of lower-back pain. The Gut Trust (now the IBS Network) noted that: 'people with IBS often report improvements with therapies such as massage, aromatherapy and acupuncture.'

In this chapter you'll find a brief overview of complementary therapies that could help ease your IBS symptoms, along with simple techniques and treatments for particular symptoms that you could try for yourself at home.

43 Apply acupressure

Acupressure is part of traditional Chinese medicine and is often described as 'acupuncture without needles'. Like acupuncture, it's based on the idea that life energy, or qi, flows through channels in the body known as meridians. An even passage of qi throughout the body is viewed as vital to good health. Disruption of the flow of qi in a meridian can lead to illness at any point within it. The flow of qi can be affected by various factors, including stress, emotional distress, diet and environment. Qi is most concentrated at points along the meridians known as acupoints. There's scientific evidence that stimulating particular acupoints can relieve both pain and nausea. Acupressure is similar to reflexology, in that it involves working on one area of the body to affect another.

The great eliminator

As the name suggests, this is thought to be good for constipation, as it is said to promote elimination.

Press your index finger and your thumb on your left hand together, and note where the webbing in between stands out the most. Now hold this point between your right thumb and index finger, applying firm pressure, having first opened the left finger and thumb. Repeat on the right hand.

44 Use aroma power

Essential oils are extracted from the petals, leaves, stalks, roots, seeds, nuts and even the bark of plants using various methods. Aromatherapy is based on the belief that, when scents released from essential oils are inhaled, they affect the hypothalamus. This is the part of the brain which governs the glands and hormones, altering mood and lowering stress. When used in massage, baths and compresses, the oils are also absorbed through the bloodstream and transported to the organs and glands, which benefit from their healing effects. Since IBS is often linked to emotional stress, aromatherapy may be worth trying, both as a preventative measure and during a flare-up.

Note

With most essential oils, use a two per cent dilution: this equates to 2 drops per teaspoon of carrier oil. A carrier oil can be any vegetable oil, including good-quality olive oil or sunflower oil, from your kitchen. Almond, sesame seed, or grapeseed oils are equally good. Never apply aromatherapy oils to broken skin.

There are various oils that may help with IBS symptoms. Some are thought to help ease diarrhoea through their calming and soothing effects on the walls of the intestine. Others are antispasmodic, which means they ease cramping, and some are carminative, which means they relieve wind. If you feel that your IBS is stress-related, there are several oils that may help you relax and ward off attacks. Studies have suggested that essential oils, such as neroli, valerian or lavender, can relieve stress by inducing relaxation and calm. Below are some other oils that are especially recommended.

Ease cramps with peppermint

We have already looked at the beneficial effects of peppermint oil when taken internally. When applied externally, it is especially good for relieving cramping. Patricia Davis, author of *Aromatherapy: An A–Z*, recommends using it well diluted (1 drop per teaspoon of carrier oil) to massage the stomach. She also advises drinking peppermint tea to intensify the effects of the massage.

Calm yourself with camomile

Camomile has been used medicinally for thousands of years. Camomile essential oil has calming effects, making it useful if your symptoms are stress-related. According to Patricia Davis, it also has anti-allergic properties, and is her first choice when food allergies are involved in your digestive problems. Try a relaxing massage using this oil (see the Massage section, p.126) or add a few drops to a warm bath to help you unwind and sleep more soundly.

Relieve symptoms with black pepper

Black pepper has been used both medicinally and as a culinary spice for over 4,000 years. Black pepper oil has a warming effect and is antispasmodic and carminative, yet also acts as a tonic and a stimulant. This means it not only soothes tummy cramps and relieves wind, but also stimulates a sluggish digestive system – making it a great all-round oil suitable for all types of IBS. Massage the diluted oil gently over your tummy area, or use it on a soothing compress.

Simply fill a basin with hot water and add a few drops of oil. Take a facecloth or handkerchief and soak it in the liquid.

Wring it out and then apply to the affected area. The heat aids absorption, provides comfort and eases pain. Other oils that you could use in this way to relieve cramps and stimulate digestion include ginger and fennel.

Try antidepressant oils

Depression is thought to be both a cause and an effect of IBS. A number of essential oils are recommended for their antidepressant qualities. These include bergamot, clary, sage, jasmine, lavender, neroli, rose, sandalwood and ylang-ylang.

45 Enjoy a massage

Massage involves touch – which can ease away stress and tension. It's thought to work by stimulating the release of endorphins (the body's own painkillers) and serotonin (a brain chemical involved in relaxation). It also decreases the level of stress hormones in the blood and improves the circulation. The IBS Network (formerly The Gut Trust) reported that many of its members noted an improvement in their IBS symptoms when they had regular massages.

Mix your own massage oil by combining 8 drops of your favourite aromatherapy oil, e.g. lavender, camomile or neroli, into 20 ml (1 tablespoon) of carrier oil, such as olive, sunflower, almond or sesame. An easy way to benefit from massage is for you and a partner to massage each other's back, neck and shoulders, using the basic techniques outlined below:

Stroking/effleurage – glide both hands over the skin in rhythmic fanning or circular motions.

Kneading – using alternate hands, squeeze and release flesh between the fingers and thumbs, as if you're kneading dough.

Friction – using your thumbs, apply even pressure to static points, or make small circles on either side of the spine.

Hacking – relax your hands then use the sides quickly and alternately to give short, sharp taps all over.

Playing some relaxing music in the background can enhance the feelings of relaxation.

46 Find relief in reflexology

Reflexology is based on the idea that points on the feet, hands and face, known as reflexes, correspond to different parts of the body (e.g. glands and organs). These are linked via vertical zones, along which energy flows. Illness occurs when these zones become blocked. Stimulating the reflexes using the fingers and thumbs is thought to bring about physiological changes which remove these blockages and encourage the mind and body to self-heal.

Practitioners believe that imbalances in the body result in granular deposits in the relevant reflex, which cause tenderness. Corns, bunions and even hard skin are all believed to indicate problems in the related parts of the body. There is no reliable evidence that reflexology relieves digestive disorders, such as IBS, but there's anecdotal evidence that reflexology foot massage is relaxing. So, at the very least, trying these techniques may relieve stress and, thus, lessen the frequency of your symptoms.

A reflexologist will usually work on your feet, because they believe the feet are more sensitive. However, it's usually easier to work on your hands when you are self-treating.

Relax an overactive gut

1. Warm your hands by rubbing the outside edges of each thumb.

2. Using a comfortable level of pressure, creep your left thumb across your right palm, in rows from left to right, starting just below the knuckle bones and finishing just above the wrist.

3. Repeat on your left hand, using your right thumb.

47 Get help with homeopathy

Homeopathy means 'same suffering' and is based on the idea that 'like cures like' – substances that can cause symptoms in a well person can treat the same symptoms in a person who is ill. For example, coffee contains caffeine, of which excessive amounts are linked to an overactive mind and insomnia, so the remedy *Coffea* is often prescribed for these very symptoms.

Symptoms like inflammation or fever are viewed as a sign that the body is trying to heal itself. The theory is that homeopathic remedies encourage this self-healing process and work in a similar way to vaccines. Homeopaths warn that there may be a worsening of symptoms at first and that this shows the body's self-healing mechanism has been stimulated.

The substances used in homeopathic remedies come from plant, animal, mineral, bark and metal sources. These substances are turned into a tincture, which is then diluted many times over. Homeopaths claim that the more diluted a remedy is, the higher its potency and the lower its potential side effects. They believe in the 'memory of water', the theory that, even though the molecules from a substance are diluted until it is unlikely that any remain, they leave behind an electromagnetic 'footprint' – like a recording on an audiotape – which still has an effect on the body.

These ideas are controversial and many GPs remain sceptical. Evidence to support homeopathy exists, but critics argue that much of it is inconclusive. For example, research published in 2005 reported improvements in symptoms and well-being among 70 per cent of patients receiving individualised homeopathy. The study involved 6,500 patients over a six-year period at the Bristol Homeopathic Hospital. However, critics of the research argue that there was no comparison group and patients may have given a positive response because it was expected. Despite this, many people claim to have been helped by homeopathy, so it may well be worth trying.

There are two main types of remedies – whole person-based and symptom-based. It's probably best to consult a qualified homeopath who will prescribe a remedy aimed at you as a whole person, based on your personality, as well as the symptoms you experience. However, if you prefer, you can buy homeopathic remedies at many high street pharmacies and health shops.

Below is a list of homeopathic remedies, along with the IBS-related physical and psychological symptoms for which they're indicated. To self-prescribe, simply choose the remedy with indications that most closely match your symptoms. Follow the dosage instructions on the product.

Argentum nitricum – for digestive upsets, such as bloating, tummy rumbling, wind, nausea, and alternating diarrhoea and constipation, linked to nervousness and anxiety.

Cantharis – particularly suitable for women and is recommended where there is inflammation of the whole digestive tract leading to burning abdominal pain, nausea and vomiting.

Carbo vegetabilis – recommended for indigestion and wind, especially when it's accompanied by chronic fatigue.

Colocynthis – for cutting pain, cramping and diarrhoea, especially when linked to unexpressed anger.

Nux vomica – recommended for abdominal pain and bowel problems with tension and irritability, particularly when applying firm pressure to the stomach brings some relief.

Sanicula aqua – for common IBS symptoms, such as bloating and belching and the need to pass stools immediately after eating.

Note

Practitioners caution people that homeopathy isn't a 'quick fix' – the remedies may take a while to take effect. Homeopathic remedies are generally considered safe and don't have any known side effects, though sometimes a temporary worsening of symptoms, known as 'aggravation' may take place. This is seen as a good sign, as it suggests that the remedy is encouraging the healing process. If this happens, stop taking the remedy and wait for your symptoms to improve. If there is steady improvement, don't restart the remedy. If the improvement stops, resume taking the remedy.

48 Try self-hypnosis

Hypnotherapists encourage a state of mind that's similar to deep daydreaming and that promotes deep relaxation and openness to suggestion. Trance-like states have been used for centuries by different cultures to encourage healing, and hypnotherapy is now quite well established as a treatment for IBS. There are two main theories on why hypnotherapy works for IBS. One is that it makes people less anxious, which somehow makes the bowel less sensitive and therefore reduces symptoms. Another explanation is that hypnotherapy may affect a part of the brain that processes pain (the anterior cingulate cortex).

Dr Peter Whorwell, Professor of Medicine and Gastroenterology in the School of Medicine at the University of Manchester, runs the hypnotherapy and irritable bowel unit at Wythenshawe Hospital in Manchester. He has spent over 20 years researching the effects of hypnotherapy on IBS.

During an interview with Dr Mark Porter on BBC Radio 4, he said: 'When thinking about irritable bowel, you have to remember there's a person round the bowel and, if that person's distressed, that bowel's going to reflect that stress.' He said there is no doubt that hypnosis helps stress, but added, 'We're pretty certain now that hypnosis does more than that and we feel that we are actually teaching the patient to control gut function.' His research suggests that the lining of the gut is much less sensitive after hypnosis and contractions, or spasms of the gut, can be reduced. He claims a success rate of 50–60 per cent with men and 70 per cent with women.

Pamela Cruickshanks, a hypnotherapist working in the unit, explained how staff there use hypnosis sessions based around imagining that the gut is like a river peacefully flowing along through beautiful countryside, and added, 'If you've got diarrhoea it's more like a waterfall and when you've got constipation it's more like the walls of the river have fallen in.'

Some self-hypnosis techniques for IBS sufferers

Most people can learn safe and simple self-hypnosis techniques. The following steps will take you through a basic self-hypnosis, which could aid relaxation and positive thinking and possibly help ease your IBS symptoms.

- Lie or sit comfortably in a quiet place, where you're unlikely to be disturbed.

- Focus on your breathing – breathe slowly and deeply.

- Start counting backwards from 300. If your mind starts to drift away, simply start counting backwards again.

- Begin relaxing each part of your body. Feel the muscles in your face relax, then those in your neck and shoulders, back, arms and legs, and finally your feet.

- Now repeat affirmations (positive statements about yourself) as though they're already true, e.g. 'I'm confident and relaxed in all situations' and 'My stomach is calm and working perfectly'. When you're ready to come out of your trance, start counting to ten, telling yourself: 'When I reach five I'll start to awaken, when I reach ten I'll wake up feeling calm and relaxed.'

49 Visualise yourself symptom-free

Visualisation involves using your imagination to create a picture of the situation you want to achieve in your mind. Using visualisation during self-hypnosis appears to improve its success and is called hypnotic imaging.

It is claimed that the more senses you use in your visualisation, the more effective it is likely to be.

Visualisation for IBS-C

Follow the self-hypnosis techniques outlined above. Then follow these steps:

1. Imagine your gut is a river, with a dam going across it, blocking its flow.

2. Next, in your mind, see the dam floating away, bit by bit, down the river.

3. Now imagine the river flowing gently and peacefully through beautiful countryside.

4. Finally, imagine a healthier, more relaxed you, free from constipation. Imagine what this healthier you looks like. Feel how much better you feel when your digestive system is working perfectly.

Visualisation for IBS-D

Follow the self-hypnosis techniques outlined above. Then follow these steps:

1. Imagine your gut is a fast-flowing river. Hear the loud roar of the water as it gushes along.

2. Next, in your mind, see the water gradually slowing down.

3. Now, imagine the river flowing slowly and gently through beautiful countryside.

4. Finally, imagine a calmer, healthier you, free from diarrhoea. Imagine what this healthier you looks like. Feel how much better you feel when your digestive system is working perfectly.

50 Say 'yes' to yoga

A study by gastroenterologists at the University of British Columbia in Vancouver suggested that yoga helps to reduce IBS symptoms. It is thought that yoga is especially beneficial because it not only exercises the body, but also relaxes the mind. The gentle stretching postures and controlled breathing exercises help release tension and reduce the effects of stress – one of the common triggers of IBS.

Useful postures

Poses claimed to be especially beneficial for IBS sufferers include the spinal twist, which strengthens the abdominal muscles, helping the colon to function more efficiently. A simple knee-to-chest pose called apanasana is thought to relieve wind and stimulate a sluggish bowel, as well as calm an overactive one. Instructions for both of these poses can be found at www.womenfitness.net/yoga_to_manage_ibs.htm.

Another pose called pavanamuktasana, from the Sanskrit words *pavana*, meaning air or wind, and *mukta*, meaning freedom or release, works on the digestive system, helping to eliminate excess gas from the stomach. For details of useful websites offering further information and guidance about yoga and yoga products, see the Directory.

However, the best and probably the most fun way to learn yoga is to attend classes run by a qualified teacher. To find one near you, go to the British Wheel of Yoga's website: www.bwy.org.uk.

Recipes

This section contains recipes based on some of the dietary recommendations outlined in chapters 2 and 3. Remember that IBS is an individual condition – foods that suit one sufferer may not suit another, so you may need to omit or replace some of the ingredients listed.

Mixed bean soup (serves four)

Beans are rich in soluble fibre, which is beneficial for most IBS sufferers. If onions exacerbate your symptoms, you could try using a small leek instead.

Ingredients
600 g mixed dried beans
1 litre vegetable stock
4 tbsp olive oil
4 celery sticks, finely chopped
2 carrots, finely chopped
1 medium onion, finely chopped
2 cloves garlic, crushed
2 sprigs rosemary
4 bay leaves
Salt and freshly ground black pepper

Method

1. Soak the beans overnight in cold water. Rinse and drain.

2. Heat the olive oil in a saucepan and gently fry the celery, carrot, onion, garlic, rosemary and bay leaves until golden.

3. Add the mixed beans and vegetable stock. Bring to the boil and simmer for 10 minutes.

4. Reduce the heat and simmer gently for about 50 minutes, or until the beans are soft.

5. Remove the rosemary sprig and bay leaves, and season with salt and freshly ground black pepper.

Salmon and leek wheat-free pasta (serves four)

This recipe contains salmon, rich in omega-3 essential fatty acids, to promote general health; leeks, to boost beneficial gut bacteria; and fennel seeds, to ease wind and cramps.

Note: this recipe can also be dairy-free if you use soya single cream and dairy-free Parmesan.

Ingredients

4 skinless and boneless salmon steaks

2 tsp fennel seeds

350 g wheat- or gluten-free pasta shapes

220 g baby leeks

400 ml single cream or soya single cream (for a dairy-free dish)

2 garlic cloves

2 tbsp extra virgin olive oil

Fresh tarragon or basil

Grated Parmesan or Parmazano (a dairy-free alternative)

Black pepper

Method

1. Preheat oven to 180°C/gas mark 4.

2. Sprinkle salmon steaks with the fennel seeds, then wrap them in tin foil and cook in oven for 15–20 minutes. Once lightly cooked, remove from oven and allow to rest.

3. Cut into 2.5 cm chunks.

4. Meanwhile, add pasta shells to large pan of boiling, lightly salted water. Bring back to the boil and cook according to instructions on the packet.

5. Chop leeks into 1 cm pieces. Wash and dry thoroughly. Heat olive oil in large frying pan until hot, turn heat to medium, add leeks and gently stir-fry for around 4 minutes.

6. Peel and crush the garlic, and add to leeks. Continue to stir-fry until the leeks are soft. Add the salmon chunks and single cream to the cooked leeks, and stir gently until mixture has heated through.

7. Add the mixture to the drained pasta and toss together with fresh tarragon or torn basil leaves.

8. Serve in pasta bowls with black pepper and Parmesan or Parmazano, to taste.

Wheat- and dairy-free banana bread

This recipe contains ripe bananas, which are thought to soothe an inflamed stomach.

Ingredients

2 medium-sized ripe bananas

150 g plain brown or white wheat-free flour

50 g dairy-free spread

10 g (2 tsp) wheat- and gluten-free baking powder

1 egg

100 ml soya milk

Method

1. Preheat the oven to 180°C/gas mark 4.

2. Place all of the ingredients in a food blender. Blend until mixture has a soft consistency.

3. Spoon the mixture into a lightly oiled loaf tin, lined with greaseproof paper.

4. Bake for about 30 minutes, or until a skewer comes out clean. Allow to cool slightly, before turning out onto a wire rack.

5. Serve thickly sliced, with a vegetable oil or soya spread.

Wheat- and gluten-free flour is available in most supermarkets. Try using white flour if you have IBS-A or IBS-D.

Wheat- and dairy-free fruit crumble

This recipe contains oats for soluble fibre, and cooked fruit, which is easier to digest than raw fruit.

Ingredients

100 g dairy-free spread
100 g demerara sugar
100 g brown or white self-raising wheat- and gluten-free flour
100 g oats
450 g any fruit – e.g. apples, plums, rhubarb or summer fruits
Sugar, to taste

Method

1. Place the fruit in an ovenproof dish. Add a little sugar to taste, if you are using a tart fruit, such as rhubarb.

2. Make the crumble by rubbing the spread into the flour until the mixture resembles breadcrumbs. Stir in the oats and demerara sugar.

3. Spread the crumble mixture over the fruit.

4. Place in an oven preheated to 180°C/gas mark 4 for 30–40 minutes, or until the crumble is golden-brown and the fruit is bubbling.

5. Serve with single cream, or soya custard.

Dairy-free apricot mousse (serves four)

This recipe contains apricots, to provide soluble fibre, and mint, to help ease wind and bloating.

Ingredients

400 g ripe, stoned apricots or dried apricots
1 packet gelatine
300 g natural soya yogurt
Sprigs fresh mint, to decorate

Method

1. Put the fresh or dried apricots in a pan. Cover with water and simmer gently for a few minutes, until soft.

2. Blend apricots into a puree.

3. Dissolve the gelatine according to the instructions on the packet.

4. Mix the apricot puree into the gelatine and then mix with the yogurt.

5. Pour into individual sundae dishes and chill until set. Decorate with sprigs of fresh mint.

Jargon Buster

A lot of literature about IBS, including this book, contains terms whose meanings you may be unclear about. Listed below are basic definitions of some of the words and phrases that might be used when discussing the diagnosis, prevention and treatment of IBS.

Anus – the opening at the end of the digestive system from which faeces (waste) leave the body.

Bile – a yellow fluid produced by the liver that is stored in the gallbladder and released to aid the digestion of fats.

Borborygmi – gurgling noises from the gut.

Carminative – a substance that prevents the formation of gas in the gut or eases its passing.

Chyme – partially digested food that has been mixed with acids in the stomach.

Duodenum – the first part of the small intestine.

Enzyme – proteins produced in the body to speed up processes like digestion.

Epiglottis – the flap at the back of the tongue that prevents chewed food from going down the windpipe to the lungs. When you swallow, your epiglottis automatically closes. When you breathe it opens, allowing air to go in and out of the windpipe.

Gall bladder – a small, sac-like organ that stores bile and releases it into the small intestine.

Gastric – literally means 'of the stomach'.

Gastric juice – fluid produced in the stomach containing hydrochloric acid and enzymes to break down food.

Gastroenterology – the study of the digestive system.

Gastrointestinal – connected to, or referring to, the stomach and intestines.

Ileum – the last part of the small intestine.

Jejunum – the middle section of the small intestine.

Laxative – something that stimulates a bowel movement – from the Latin word *Laxare*, meaning to open, widen, or release.

Liver – a large organ, situated above and in front of the stomach, that filters toxins from the blood and makes bile to break down fats.

Malfermentation – abnormal fermentation of food by 'bad' bacteria, which results in the release of toxic waste and gases.

Mouth – the first part of the digestive system, where food enters the body. Chewing and salivary enzymes in the mouth are the start of digestion.

Mucilage – a jelly-like substance produced by plants.

Mucosa – a moist membrane that secretes mucus.

Oesophagus – the long tube that uses rhythmic muscle movements (peristalsis) to push food from the throat down into the stomach.

Oestrogen – a female hormone involved in stimulating the growth of the womb lining.

Pancreas – a gland just below the stomach and above the intestines that produces enzymes to aid digestion.

Peristalsis – involuntary rhythmic muscle movements that push food along the oesophagus from the throat down into the stomach.

Prebiotics – natural indigestible starches that feed and encourage the growth of existing 'good' bacteria in the gut.

Probiotics – literally means 'for life'. Beneficial bacteria found in foods, such as natural yogurt, which are thought to aid digestion.

Progesterone – literally means 'for pregnancy'. Female hormone involved in the preparation of the womb for pregnancy.

Prostaglandins – hormone-like chemicals produced in the body to create a number of effects, including the stimulation of contractions in the uterus and other smooth muscle.

Receptors – proteins on the surface of cells designed to bind with and react to specific substances in the body, e.g. hormones and insulin.

Rectum – the lower part of the large intestine, where faeces are stored before they are expelled from the body.

Saliva – fluid produced by salivary glands containing enzymes that break down carbohydrates (starch) into smaller molecules.

Salivary glands – glands located in the mouth that produce saliva.

Stomach – a sack-like, muscular organ that is attached to the oesophagus, and where both chemical and mechanical digestion takes place.

Useful Products

Below is a list of products and suppliers of products that may help ease the symptoms of IBS. The author doesn't endorse or recommend any particular product and this list is by no means exhaustive.

Bimuno Powder
Supplement containing prebiotics and probiotics to help boost beneficial bacteria in the gut.
  Website: www.bimuno.com

Cynara Artichoke
A supplement containing 320 mg of standardised artichoke leaf dry extract per capsule to help maintain a healthy digestive system.
  Website: www.hollandandbarrett.com

FemmeVit
A supplement containing vitamins, minerals and herbs to help regulate hormones and reduce tiredness and fatigue – including B vitamins, magnesium, chromium, starflower oil, and agnus castus.
  Website: www.healthaid.co.uk

IBS Hypnosis

A guided self-hypnosis session, available as an MP3 download or as a CD, that aims to help you change the way your body feels by using your unconscious mind to relax your stomach, reducing discomfort and bloating.

Website: www.selfhypnosis.com/downloads/ibs-management

Imodium IBS Relief

Easy-to-swallow capsules that contain loperamide and are specifically designed to relieve IBS-related diarrhoea quickly. Available in pharmacies and supermarkets nationwide.

Website: www.imodium.co.uk

J. L. Bragg's Medicinal Charcoal

Activated charcoal has been clinically proven to relieve wind and bloating. Available in biscuit, powder, tablet or capsule form.

Website: www.charcoal.uk.com

Lepicol

A supplement that may help all types of IBS, containing ispaghula husks, prebiotics (fructo-oligosaccharides) and the probiotics *Lactobacillus* and bifidobacteria. One sachet is taken twice daily, mixed with water or fruit juice. This product is wheat- and gluten-free and suitable for vegans.

Website: www.lepicol.com

Multibionta

A multivitamin and mineral supplement containing three probiotics – one strain of *Lactobacillus* and two of *Bifidobacterium*. The tablets are enteric-coated to prevent stomach acids from destroying the probiotics. It is reasonably priced and available in five different formulas to suit different age groups and lifestyles.

Website: www.multibionta.co.uk

Ortis Fruits & Fibres Chewable Cubes

Chewable fruit-flavoured cubes containing figs, senna and natural orange extract to ease constipation.

Website: www.hollandandbarrett.com

Pukka Detox

A herbal tea with aniseed, cardamom, coriander, fennel, licorice and celery seeds to relax the digestive system and reduce bloating.

Website: www.pukkaherbs.com

Pukka Relax

A relaxing tea that calms and relieves bloating. Contains organic camomile, licorice root, fennel seeds, ginger, marshmallow root, oat flowering tops and cardamom pods.

Website: www.pukkaherbs.com

RADAR key

A key that can unlock disabled toilets across the UK that are part of the National Key Scheme run by Disability Rights UK. You can buy a RADAR key from the charity's website.

Website: crm.disabilityrightsuk.org/radar-nks-key

Senokot

Senokot is a range of products that contain the laxative senna. Senokot tablets and syrup start to work 8 to 12 hours after you take them, and should be taken at night to relieve constipation the following morning. Senokot Dual Relief also contains fennel to relieve bloating.

Website: www.senokot.co.uk

Solgar Calcium Citrate with Vitamin D3

A supplement containing calcium citrate, the most easily absorbed form of calcium. Also contains vitamin D3 to aid calcium absorption.

Website: www.solgar.co.uk

Symprove

A gluten- and dairy-free multi-probiotic drink that contains four live bacteria: *L. rhamnosus*, *E. faecium*, *L. acidophilus*, and *L. plantarum*.

Website: www.symprove.com

Tisserand Aromatherapy

This company offers a wide range of good quality essential oils designed to improve health and happiness.

Website: www.tisserand.com

Helpful Books

Brewer, Dr Sarah and Berriedale-Johnson, Michelle *The IBS Diet* (Thorsons, 2004) – a useful book containing a wide range of recipes, including high- and low-fibre, and gluten- and lactose-free dishes, to suit the diverse dietary needs of IBS sufferers.

Carlson, Richard, *Don't Sweat the Small Stuff... and It's All Small Stuff: Simple ways to keep the little things from taking over your life* (Mobius, 1998) – this book offers some effective strategies to help you achieve inner calm.

Carlson, Richard, *Stop Thinking, Start Living: Discover lifelong happiness* (Element, 1997) – this book explains how happiness is a state of mind and is not dependent on circumstances.

Shepherd, Dr Sue and Gibson, Dr Peter *The Complete Low-FODMAP Diet: The revolutionary plan for managing symptoms in IBS, Crohn's disease, coeliac disease and other digestive disorders* (Vermilion, 2014) – the definitive guide to the low-FODMAP diet written by the nutritionist and gastroenterologist who developed it.

Shepherd, Dr Sue, *The Low-FODMAP Diet Cookbook: 150 simple and delicious recipes to relieve symptoms of IBS, Crohn's disease, coeliac disease and other digestive disorders* (Vermilion, 2015)

– contains a wide range of recipes that are gluten-free and low in the sugars that can cause IBS symptoms. Includes ideas for breakfast, light bites, main meals and desserts.

Smith Sinclair, Carol *The IBS Low-Starch Diet: Why starchy food may be hazardous to your health* (Vermilion, 2006) – this book outlines how the author overcame IBS and arthritis by following a starch-free diet. It includes over 200 starch- and gluten-free recipes and may be worth reading if you have tried other dietary and lifestyle changes and conventional treatments without success. However, it is strongly recommended that you seek advice from your GP or dietician before following any of the dietary changes suggested in this book.

Directory

The following list of contacts offers information and support for IBS sufferers.

ABC of Yoga

A website offering tips, advice and step-by-step animated posture guides for those who wish to practise yoga at home. Also provides meditation techniques.

Website: www.abc-of-yoga.com

Allergy UK (formerly The British Allergy Foundation)

A nationwide medical charity for people with allergies, food intolerances and chemical sensitivities. Provides up-to-date information on all aspects of allergies, including the different symptoms caused by food intolerance, such as IBS, and how to identify what might be causing them.

Website: www.allergyuk.org

Better Digestive Health

A website from McNeil Products Limited (manufacturers of Imodium) with useful information about the digestive system and digestive disorders, including IBS.

Website: www.imodium.co.uk

Bladder and Bowel Foundation

Formerly known as Incontact and the Continence Foundation, this is the UK's leading charity for information and support for people with bladder and bowel disorders – including IBS – their carers, families and healthcare professionals.

Website: www.bladderandbowelfoundation.org

British Wheel of Yoga

The national governing body for yoga in the UK, with a nationwide network of over 3,000 teachers.

Website: www.bwy.org.uk

CORE

A digestive health charity offering evidence-based information on a wide range of digestive disorders, including IBS.

Website: www.corecharity.org.uk

Foods Matter

An independent website that offers information on food allergies and intolerances and up-to-date information on the latest research.

Website: www.foodsmatter.com

Help for IBS

A site run by American IBS sufferer and expert Heather Van Vorous that offers information, recipes and helpful products for IBS, such as herbal teas and self-hypnosis CDs. You can also access message boards and details of support groups.

Website: www.helpforibs.com

The Henry Spink Foundation

An independent charity created to help families of children with severe disabilities of all kinds, providing information on conventional and alternative medicine, therapies and research relating to a wide range of physical and mental disorders. Includes a large section on candida, which some people believe is implicated in some cases of IBS.

Website: www.henryspink.org

The IBS Network

A UK charity for IBS sufferers (formerly known as The Gut Trust) that offers general information on IBS on its website. If you become a member you will have access to a medical helpline staffed by specialist nurses, fact sheets, recipes, online expert advice and support, toilet access cards, as well as a quarterly journal, monthly newsletter, internet forums, a network of self-help groups and a self-management programme. Online membership costs £24 annually and postal membership costs £34 a year. Medical helpline (members only) is open 7 p.m.–9 p.m. on Tuesdays, Wednesdays and Thursdays.

Website: www.theibsnetwork.org

IBS Relief

A website sponsored by the makers of the antispasmodic drug Buscopan. Offers some useful information and advice for IBS sufferers, including a downloadable IBS diary app and video clips demonstrating how to do helpful yoga exercises.

Website: www.ibs-relief.co.uk

IBS Tales

A site where IBS sufferers can tell their stories as well as read about others' experiences. There is also general information about IBS and reviews of IBS medications, diets, supplements and therapies.

Website: www.ibstales.com

Irritable Bowel Syndrome Self Help and Support Group

A US online self-help and support group for IBS sufferers. As well as forums and blogs, the site offers up-to-date information about the condition.

Website: www.ibsgroup.org

Love Your Gut

A website offering information and advice on gut health, including diet and lifestyle tips and gut-friendly recipes.

Website: www.loveyourgut.com

Medicines and Healthcare products Regulatory Agency (MHRA)

A government agency responsible for ensuring that medicines and medical devices work and are safe.

Website: www.mhra.gov.uk

Mind

A national charity for people with emotional and mental health problems. Offers advice online and through a network of local Mind associations that offer counselling, befriending and drop-in sessions, etc.

Website: www.mind.org.uk

Relaxation for Living Institute

Offers courses, DVDs and CDs that aim to teach people how to relax and deal with stress and anxiety using breathing- and muscle-relaxation techniques.

Website: www.rfli.co.uk

Shepherd Works

Website providing information on the low-FODMAP diet from Dr Sue Shepherd, the nutritionist who helped develop it in 1999.

Website: www.shepherdworks.com.au

The Stress Management Society

The Stress Management Society is a non-profit-making organisation dedicated to helping people tackle stress. Website offers information on stress-management techniques, such as self-hypnosis and self-massage. The society also offers a free e-newsletter, an online stress coaching tool and stress-management workshops.

Website: www.stress.org.uk

Tummy Trouble

Website that aims to provide information on stomach and abdominal aches and pains, and their causes, symptoms and relief.

Website: www.tummytrouble.co.uk

Yoga Abode

An online magazine and community for yoga fans. Offers technical advice on yoga postures and yoga products, as well as a directory of yoga classes, workshops and retreats.

Website: www.yoga-abode.com

Yoga 2 Hear

A website offering CD and MP3 hatha yoga class downloads, suitable for all levels and abilities, including a free 'taster session'.

www.yoga2hear.co.uk

Have you enjoyed this book?
If so, why not write a review on your favourite website?

If you're interested in finding out more about our books, find
us on Facebook at **Summersdale Publishers** and follow us on
Twitter at **@Summersdale**.

Thanks very much for buying this Summersdale book.

www.summersdale.com